ABC OF NUTRITION

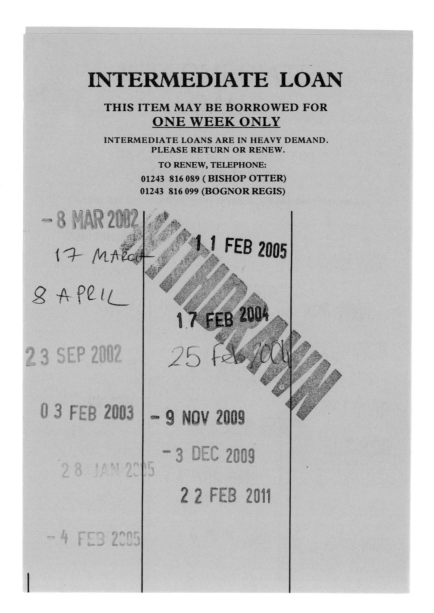
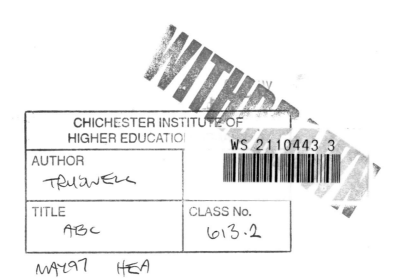

ABC OF NUTRITION
SECOND EDITION

A STEWART TRUSWELL MD FRCP FFPHM

Boden Professor of Human Nutrition
University of Sydney

with contributions from

JANETTE C BRAND MILLER, MILES IRVING, NORMAN D NOAH

Published by the British Medical Journal
Tavistock Square, London WC1H 9JR

First Edition 1986
Second Impression 1987
Third Impression 1989
Fourth Impression 1989
Second Edition 1992
Second Impression 1992
Fourth Impression 1994

British Library Cataloguing in Publication Data

Truswell, A. Stewart
  ABC of Nutrition–2nd ed
  I. Title
  614.5939

ISBN 0 7279 0315 2

Printed in England by Eyre & Spottiswoode Ltd,
London and Margate
Typesetting by Apek Typesetters, Nailsea, Bristol

Preface to the Second Edition

I was asked to write the original series of ABC articles on nutrition for an imagined general practitioner who had been taught almost no nutrition at medical school and now felt the need for it in the practice but could spare only about 15 minutes a week for this reading. Other instructions were to use nearly half the page (the left half) for illustrations and to write without references and that the writing had to be practical.

The original articles appeared in the BMJ in 1985. Each article was about nutrition in different clinical settings. With no discouraging basic biochemistry we plunged straight into the common question of diet and coronary heart disease. We didn't come to "some principles" until the last article.

As the articles appeared, specialists wrote to the journal; letters published in the correspondence pages suggested corrections of detail or of wording. All these were used to revise the articles when each became a chapter in the ABC book, first published by the BMJ in 1986.

One of the problems with nutrition is that it is often presented in a theoretical and passive way. I have tried in the ABC to emphasise the active and practical aspects. Reviews of the first edition were very encouraging and I have responded to any justified criticisms. The book has been popular among doctors, medical students, nurses, dentists, and other health professionals; it has been adopted in many medical schools and has been translated into Spanish and Italian.

In this second edition the text has been updated throughout. The text has been expanded where it appeared too brief, and some references have been provided for people who like to read further. Chapters that were originally double articles, on the Third World, vitamins, and obesity, have been consolidated, and the order of chapters is more systematic.

This book does not deal with all aspects of human nutrition, only those that are useful in medical practice. The latest fads and controversies are not here either. This is the ABC of Nutrition, not the XYZ.

A STEWART TRUSWELL
January 1992

Many of the ideas in this ABC came from discussions over the years with colleagues, of whom the following have helped towards the writing of one or more of the chapters: Ms Marianne Sylvada de Soza; Professors P J V Beaumont, John Garrow, J G A J Hautvast, M Katan, J I Mann, B E C Nordin, and Dave Roberts; Drs Margaret Allman, Susan Ash, Janette Brand Miller, Trevor Beard, David Buss, Cathie Hull, Rob Loblay, Peter Roeser, Samir Samman, Anne Swain, Anne Thorburn, Clive West, and Debbie Zador; and Mr K J Dale.

Contents

1: REDUCING THE RISK OF CORONARY HEART DISEASE

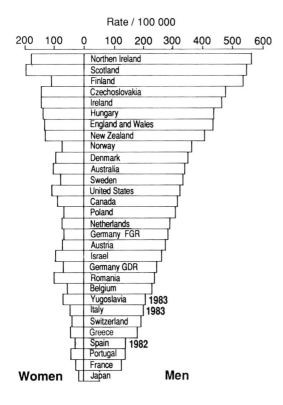

Rate / 100 000

Coronary heart disease, the leading cause of death in Britain and other Western countries, is only one tenth as common in industrial Japan and rare in most Third World communities. Its incidence is environmentally determined because immigrant groups soon take on the incidence of their host country and there have been large changes over time in mortality from coronary heart disease. It was uncommon before 1925 and then rose steadily except for a dip in Europe in the second world war. Age standardised mortality rates from coronary heart disease in the United States and Australia have come down by more than 50% since their peak in the mid 1960s. Smaller reductions have occurred in Finland, New Zealand, Canada, The Netherlands, and Belgium. In Britain coronary mortality was static until about 1980, since when it has slowly declined. Rates are higher in Northern Ireland and Scotland, and in 1985 and 1986 these two parts of the United Kingdom had the highest coronary mortalities in the world, in men and women. In the countries of eastern Europe (Czechoslovakia, Hungary, Poland, Bulgaria, and the USSR), meanwhile, coronary mortalities have been rising.

Coronary heart disease mortality for men and women aged 40–69 (age standardised rates/ 100 000 for 1985 unless otherwise stated)[1]

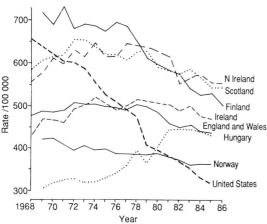

Trends in coronary heart disease mortality for men aged 40–69, 1968–89 (age adjusted rates/100 000 for certain countries)[1]

Coronary heart disease is a multifactorial disease, but diet is probably the fundamental environmental factor. The pathological basis is atherosclerosis, which takes years to develop. Thrombosis superimposed on an atherosclerotic plaque, which takes hours, usually precipitates a clinical event. Then whether the patient dies suddenly, has a classic myocardial infarct, develops angina, or has asymptomatic electrocardiographic changes depends on the state of the myocardium. Each of these three processes is likely to be affected by different components in the diet.

Atherosclerosis and cholesterol

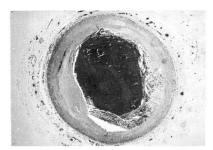

Photomicrograph of coronary artery with atherosclerosis

The characteristic material that accumulates in atherosclerosis is cholesterol. This and other lipids in the plaque come from the blood, where they are carried on lipoproteins. In animals atheroma can be produced by raising plasma cholesterol concentrations with high fat diets.

People with familial increases in low density lipoprotein (LDL) cholesterol (familial hypercholesterolaemia) tend to have premature coronary heart disease: this is accelerated even more in homozygotes, who all develop clinical coronary heart disease before they are 20.

Reducing the risk of coronary heart disease

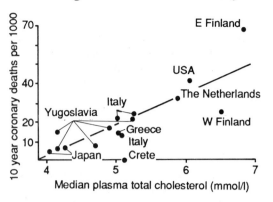

Plasma cholesterol related to deaths from coronary heart disease during 10 years in 16 communities in the seven country prospective study (correlation coefficient + 0·8)[2]

Over 20 prospective studies in 14 countries all show that high plasma LDL (or total) cholesterol, arterial hypertension, and cigarette smoking are the big three risk factors for coronary heart disease.

The mean plasma total cholesterol of healthy adults ranges widely in different communities, from 3·0 mmol/l in Bushmen and Masai to 7·2 mmol/l in east Finland a few years ago. None of the other common biochemical plasma variables show this variation. Only in countries whose average total cholesterol exceeds 5·2 mmol/l (200 mg/dl)—as in Britain—is coronary heart disease common.

Some countries where expert committes have recommended reductions in plasma cholesterol
Australia
Canada
Finland
The Netherlands
New Zealand
Norway
Sweden
United Kingdom
United States
Germany

Individuals at increased risk
Family history of coronary heart disease
Plasma cholesterol >6·5 mmol/l
Hypertension
Smoking
Obesity
Angina
ECG abnormalities
Diabetes

Countries at increased risk—A major strategy of primary prevention for a whole country—or for the people in a district, or even in a practice—is to advise people to modify their diet to achieve a modest reduction in plasma total cholesterol. This can be done gently and inexpensively.

Individuals at increased risk—For individuals at increased risk of coronary heart disease a stricter cholesterol lowering diet should be prescribed, and drugs may be indicated if hypercholesterolaemia does not fall satisfactorily.

Doctor, please take my blood for cholesterol measurement. Then what?

Suggested action[3][4] if initial plasma concentration is about 6·5 mmol/l:
1 Patient to fast overnight
2 Take blood sample for **repeat** test
If confirmed plasma *total* cholesterol is:
5·2 to 6·5 mmol/l:
Advise on weight reduction if patient's body mass index (BMI) is above 25
Recommend reduced saturated fat diet
6·5 to 7·8 mmol/l:
Give serious dietary advice (see box on next page) and follow up
Help of a dietitian valuable
Check and deal with associated coronary risk factors, eg smoking, hypertension
Encouragement and cooperation of patient's spouse important for compliance
Check response to diet by repeating plasma cholesterol (preferably fasting) after three or four weeks
Consider drug treatment if response to diet is poor
7·8 mmol/l or more:
Repeat fasting blood test (again) for cholesterol, and test for HDL and triglyceride
Consider referral to hyperlipidaemia clinic

The risk of coronary disease increases progressively with plasma cholesterol.[5][6] Many sets of data show that people with higher concentrations than 6·5 mmol/l (250 mg/dl) are at high risk. People with plasma cholesterol between 5·2 mmol/l (200 mg/dl) and 6·5 mmol/l are at moderate risk. High cholesterols seem to have the greatest effect in young adults and little effect in old people.

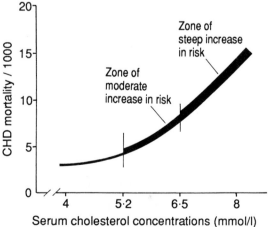

Relation between serum (total) cholesterol and risk of coronary heart disease (CHD)[5] based on a six years follow up of over 350 000 middle aged men in the United States.[6]

Fatty acid patterns of fats, oils, and some meats (as % total fat in the food)

| | Saturated | | | | | |
	C4–12	C14–18 (myristic, palmitic, stearic)	Mono-unsaturated	Linoleic	Other poly-unsaturated	P:S*
Butter, cream, milk	13	48	30	**2**	1	0·05
Cocoa butter	—	61	36	**3**	—	0·05
Beef	—	48	48	**2**	1	0·06
Coconut oil	58	31	8	**2**	—	0·1
Bacon and pork	—	42	50	**7**	1	0·2
Palm oil (used in ice cream)	—	45	45	**9**	—	0·2
Margarine (old style, hard)	3	37	33	**12**	1	0·3
Chicken	—	34	45	**18**	2	0·6
Olive oil	—	14	73	**11**	1	0·9
Groundnut oil	—	15	53	**30**	1	2·1
Fish oil	—	23	27	**7**	43†	2·2
Margarine, polyunsaturated	2	21	22	**52**	1	2·3
Corn (maize) oil	—	14	24	**53**	2	3·9
Soya bean oil	—	14	24	**53**	7	4·3
Canola oil	—	7	63	**20**	10‡	4·3
Sunflower seed oil	—	12	33	**58**	—	4·8

* These are in ascending order of ratio of polyunsaturated to saturated fats, but this is not the only consideration in choosing dietary fats and oils.
† Includes varying amounts of eicosapentenaenoic acid (20:5, ω − 3) (depending on species).
‡ α Linolenic acid

In Britain many people, more than 50% of adults, have plasma cholesterols above 5·2 mmol/l, and about 25% have concentrations above 6·5 mmol/l.[5 7]

Principles of cholesterol-lowering diet

Fat—The major dietary influence on plasma LDL and total cholesterol is the amount and type of fat. The elevating effect comes mostly from saturated fatty acids, palmitic and myristic. (There is more palmitic in most diets.) Polyunsaturated fats, chiefly linoleic acid, tend to lower plasma LDL and total cholesterol but their effect is only half as strong as the elevating effect of palmitic acid. Monounsaturated fats, chiefly oleic acid, have a somewhat smaller cholesterol-lowering effect. These effects take about 10 to 14 days to appear and last for years provided that people stick to the diet.

Dietary cholesterol—Other dietary components have smaller effects. Lay people and the media confuse dietary cholesterol with plasma cholesterol. Eating cholesterol or eggs (the richest common source of cholesterol) in general has less effect on plasma cholesterol values than eating saturated fats, and some people are more sensitive than others.

Diet with reduced saturated fat and cholesterol, partially replaced by polyunsaturated fat, to lower plasma cholesterol (total and LDL)

Sample daily menu

Breakfast: Grapefruit or orange juice
Cereal or oatmeal porridge with skim milk
Toast, polyunsaturated margarine, and marmalade or jam
Coffee or tea with skim milk (and sugar)

Mid-morning: Coffee or tea with skim milk (and sugar)

Lunch: Sandwiches made from bread and polyunsaturated margarine and filled with sardines, tuna, salmon, tomato, cucumber, Marmite, etc
Salad (no dressing)
Fruit
Tea with skim milk (and sugar)

Mid-afternoon Tea with skim milk; piece of fruit

Dinner: Cooked poultry, fish, or lean meat, which may be stewed or grilled or fried in a little unsaturated oil
Boiled or baked potatoes *or* rice *or* pasta
Vegetables, raw or cooked
Alcoholic drink if desired
Bread or plain roll
Fruit salad or allowed dessert
Coffee with skim milk (and sugar)

Bedtime: Tea with skim milk *or* juice

General guidelines

- Avoid butter and hydrogenated margarine, lard, and suet. Use moderate amounts of polyunsaturated margarines (P:S 2 or 3).
- Avoid cream and ice cream. Use skim or semiskim (2% fat) milk instead of standard, full cream milk.
- Eat less meat and more poultry (not the skin) and fish. Choose lean meat and remove visible fat. Grill rather than fry. Avoid sausages and meat pies.
- Reduce egg yolks, visible and in recipes.
- Keep cheese intake down. Use cottage cheeses.
- Restrict intake of cakes, pastries, and biscuits (unless made at home with polyunsaturated fats), and chocolates.
- Use "unsaturated" (not just "vegetable") oils for cooking—for example, maize or sunflower oils.
- Eat more vegetables and fruits of all kinds.
- Cereals and products ad lib (bread, rice, pasta, breakfast cereals, oatmeal) and tapioca, cornflour, and sago.

Reducing the risk of coronary heart disease

Reduced energy intake—Loss of weight from reduced energy (calorie) intake can lower plasma cholesterol concentrations, especially in overweight people with an increase in both plasma cholesterol and triglycerides. But this response is not always seen: in anorexia nervosa the plasma cholesterol is often raised.

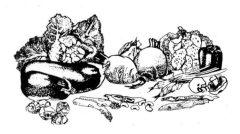

Vegetables and fruit provide vitamins, minerals, and dietary fibre. Vary the types of fruits and vegetables.

Eat four servings—select one serving which is dark green, yellow, or orange, such as leafy greens, broccoli, carrots, pumpkin, apricots, rockmelon, mangoes. Select one serving from citrus, tropical, or berry fruits, or tomatoes. Then select two servings or more of any other vegetables or fruits.

Taken from Australian dietary guidelines (modified)

Dietary fibre—The effect of dietary fibre depends on the type. Wheat fibre (bran or wholemeal bread) does not decrease plasma cholesterol values but viscous ("soluble") types, like pectin and guar, in large doses produce moderate reductions. Even 5 g/day may reduce cholesterol concentrations by about 5%. Vegetables and fruits contain around 1% pectin, and so four portions would provide about 5 g/day. Oatmeal, oat bran, and legumes all contain some soluble fibre. Generous intakes can help to lower plasma cholesterol. These foods are also likely to displace foods containing fat.

Plasma high density lipoprotein (HDL) cholesterol

High density lipoprotein (HDL) cholesterol in the plasma is a protective factor. It helps to mobilise cholesterol deposits from the tissues. HDL does not explain the big differences between countries; its mean concentration is not higher in countries with little coronary heart disease. But in countries with a high incidence of coronary heart disease individuals with above average HDL have a reduced risk. Dietary fats have small effects on HDL. Concentrations of these lipoproteins are higher in women than men, decreased in obesity, and increased by alcohol consumption.

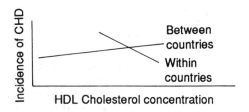

Relation of HDL cholesterol to incidence of coronary heart disease[8]

Thrombosis

The effects of diet on thrombosis can be studied only indirectly: in animals, epidemiologically, or by measuring components of the process in blood samples taken from patients, such as platelet stickiness, clotting factor concentrations, or fibrinolysis.

Eicosapentenaenoic acid (20:5, ω-3) and related very long chain marine polyunsaturated fats are the most potent inhibitors of thrombosis found in ordinary diets. Eicosapentenaenoic acid appears to act as a competitive antagonist of thromboxane A_2 formation. It is found in fatty fish like pilchards and mackerel (and fish body oils) and may explain the Eskimos' freedom from thrombotic diseases. A prospective study in Holland and a controlled trial in Cardiff both suggested that a modest intake of fatty fish (two or three times a week) may help to prevent coronary disease.[9]

Fish body oils (eg Maxepa) lower raised plasma triglyceride and tend to inhibit thrombosis. Possible side effects include bleeding and an anti-inflammatory action. They belong more with pharmacology than nutrition.

Other polyunsaturated oils—those found in seed oils like linoleic acid—have a smaller inhibiting effect on thrombosis.

High fat meals (and lipaemia) favour thrombosis and so does a high plasma cholesterol concentration.

There are scattered reports suggesting that individual foods may promote fibrinolysis—for example, onions—or inhibit it—for example, fats—but a systematic re-examination of this topic is overdue.

It seems likely that diets which reduce the tendency to thrombosis may be similar in some ways—for example, low in saturated fat—and different in others from those that lower plasma cholesterol. We know much less about the former but their potential importance is that they might reduce the risk of a first or a recurrent coronary attack after being eaten for only a few days. The best diet to prevent coronary heart disease in young adults is one that lowers plasma LDL, but in someone who already has manifest coronary disease and in old people the best diet—which now we can only see through a glass darkly—is one that makes thrombosis less likely.

Myocardium

Most unrefined foods provide moderate amounts of potassium and magnesium. There are no rich sources of potassium. Potatoes are about the best, and legumes. Meat, fish, fruit, and vegetables all provide moderate amounts of potassium.

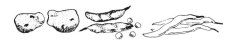

Magnesium occurs in moderate amounts in cereals (preferably wholegrain) and vegetables (in the chlorophyll). Fats and sugar contain negligible amounts of both elements.

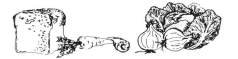

The myocardium is more susceptible to damage, prone to arrhythmias, and sensitive to digoxin in patients with low plasma potassium concentrations. It has been suggested that sudden death after exercise might sometimes be due to the plasma potassium lowering action of catecholamines. More chronic hypokalaemia is usually secondary to increased losses—for example, from diuretics. An increased potassium diet may help in such potassium losing states, but hypokalaemia is rarely due to primary dietary deficiency.

Magnesium depletion likewise is nearly always due to abnormal losses—for example, through prolonged diarrhoea, malabsorption, excessive lactation, diabetic ketoacidosis, or thiazide diuretics. Hypomagnesaemia is usually accompanied by hypocalcaemia or hypokalaemia, or both. Patients with it are liable to various fast cardiac arrhythmias and it has been reported that a minority of patients presenting with acute myocardial infarction and ventricular arrhythmias had hypomagnesaemia.

Drinking water—Total cardiovascular mortality has, as a rule, been found to be lower in districts where the drinking water is hard than in soft water areas. In Britain the latter are mostly in the old industrial areas of the north and west so it is difficult to disentangle socioeconomic factors. If the water effect is real no component has been consistently associated in different countries. Calcium appeared protective in a large British study, not magnesium. The opposite was found in a large Canadian study. The only practical conclusion as yet is that people in hard water districts would be better not to install water softeners for their drinking water.

Coronary heart disease is not an inevitable consequence of either aging or industrialisation. It appears to be largely preventable and the World Health Organisation recommends preventive community action in countries with a high incidence. The role of personal physicians is vital here. Through talking to patients and by personal example and leadership they play a major part in increasing public awareness and in modifying attitudes and behaviour that affect health.

The most active of the prevention programmes in Britain is Heartbeat Wales. This has been running since 1985 with an interdisciplinary team based in Cardiff. Initiatives in the nutrition aspect have included: food labelling in supermarkets (eg, Tesco); promoting lean meat and low fat milk, Heartbeat awards to restaurants, television programmes, dissemination of curriculum materials to schools, and a bilingual policy. Their headquarters address is: Heartbeat Wales, Ty George Thomas, 24 Park Place, Cardiff CF1 3BA.

North Karelia

North Karelia is the most easterly county of Finland. In 1971 it had the highest (age standardised) death rate from coronary disease in the world. The people were worried and asked the government for help. A community programme was set up. Everyone was advised to stop smoking, eat less fat and more vegetables, avoid obesity, and have their blood pressure checked. By 1979 coronary mortality had fallen by 24% in men and 51% in the women, a significantly greater fall than the general decline in coronary deaths in Finland during the same period.

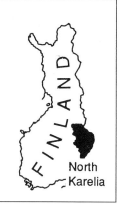

North Karelia

1 National Forum for Coronary Heart Disease Prevention. *Coronary heart disease prevention: action in the UK 1984–1987.* London: Health Education Authority, 1988.
2 Keys A. *Seven countries: a multivariate analysis of death and coronary heart disease.* Cambridge, Massachusetts: Harvard University Press, 1980.
3 Study group, European Atherosclerosis Society. Strategies for the prevention of coronary heart disease: a policy statement of the European Atherosclerosis Society. *Eur Heart J* 1987;8:77–88.
4 Lewis B, Assmann G, Mancini M, *et al. Handbook of coronary heart disease prevention.* London: Current Medical Literature, 1989.
5 Ball M, Mann JI. *Lipids and heart disease. A practical approach.* Oxford: Oxford Medical Publications, 1988.
6 Martin MJ, Hulley SB, Browner WS, Kuller LH, Wentworth D. Serum cholesterol, blood pressure and mortality: implications from a cohort of 361 662 men. *Lancet* 1986;ii:933–6.
7 Tunstall-Pedoe H, Smith WCS, Tavendale R. How-often-that-high graphs of serum cholesterol. Findings from the Scottish Heart Health and Scottish MONICA studies. *Lancet* 1989;i:540–2.
8 Knuiman JT, West CE. Differences in HDL cholesterol between populations: no paradox? *Lancet* 1983;i:296.
9 Burr ML, Fehily AM, Gilbert JF, *et al.* Effects of changes in fat, fish and fibre intakes on death and myocardial reinfarction: diet and reinfarction trial (DART). *Lancet* 1989;ii:757–61.

Further reading

Department of Health and Social Security. *Report of the Committee on Medical Aspects of Food policy: diet and cardiovascular disease.* London: HMSO, 1984.

2: DIET AND HYPERTENSION

Causal factors in essential hypertension

Genetic—several mechanisms

Tension from anxiety—via increased sympathetic tone or circulating catecholamines

Dietary—positive correlation	*—negative correlation*
Overweight and obesity	Potassium
Sodium (salt) intake	? Calcium
Alcohol	Fish oil

Essential hypertension is a multifactorial disease. It is common not only in urban and industrialised people but prevalent too in a quiet Hebridean island; in tropical Africa, where Albert Schweizer used to work; and in a Solomon Islands tribe, minimally influenced by Western ways, which cooks in sea water.

Sodium (Na)

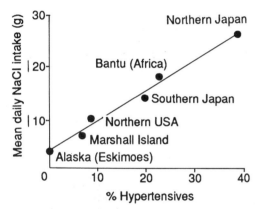

Salt intake and hypertension in various communities[2]

- Between countries the prevalence of hypertension correlates with mean salt intake

- Normotensive and hypertensive individuals usually show a fall in blood pressure when salt intake is reduced

- Individuals tend to show a small rise in blood pressure when sodium intake is increased experimentally

- Correlation of blood pressure and salt intake is often not demonstrable between individuals

When sodium accumulates in the body some goes into the smooth muscle cells of arterioles. This increases their tone and consequently the arterial blood pressure

To what extent is essential hypertension caused by an unnecessarily high intake of salt?

There are a few isolated communities in which hypertension is not seen, such as the Yanomamo Indians (in the Amazon), Kalahari Bushmen (Botswana),[1] and remote Pacific islanders. These people have very low salt (NaCl) intakes, about 2 g a day or less. In northern Japan salt intakes are very high, 25 g a day, and the incidence of hypertension and stroke is higher than in the United Kingdom.

Inability to show a consistent correlation between individual salt intake (most conveniently assessed by 24 hour urinary sodium excretion) and blood pressure is the major weakness of the salt hypothesis. Rats show genetic variations in sensitivity of blood pressure to salt intake and the same probably occurs in man. Correlation has been found in people with a family history of hypertension.

There have been several reports that people with hypertension tend to have increased sodium concentrations in cells and abnormal activities in blood cell membranes of the several mechanisms for keeping sodium out of and potassium inside the cells.

The physiological requirement for sodium (Na) is no more than 20 mmol a day, equivalent to about 1 g of salt (NaCl).

Sodium loss through the skin is very small unless there is much sweating. But people on low sodium intakes and those who have adapted to hot climates lose less sodium in sweat, about 30 mmol/l. The average salt intake in Britain is about 9 g a day (150 mmol sodium). Before the advent of canning, deep freezers, refrigerators, etc, many types of food had to be salted to preserve them. Most of mankind has therefore become used to the taste of far more salt than we need nowadays. Though a high salt intake has not yet been proved to be a cause of hypertension, substantial reductions of our salt intake can do no harm.

For the general adult population, mainly as a measure to reduce hypertension, the United States and Australia and the WHO Expert Committee on Prevention of Coronary Heart Disease (1981) recommend that people should not eat more than 6 g salt a day. The DHSS report *Diet and Cardiovascular Disease* recommends that consideration be given to ways of decreasing salt intake.[3]

Dietary goal for most adults: less than 100 mmol Na = 2·3 g Na = 6 g NaCl

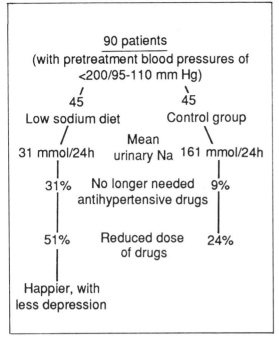

90 patients
(with pretreatment blood pressures of
<200/95-110 mm Hg)

45 — Low sodium diet   45 — Control group

31 mmol/24h — Mean urinary Na — 161 mmol/24h

31%   No longer needed antihypertensive drugs   9%

51%   Reduced dose of drugs   24%

Happier, with less depression

Trial of low salt diet in people with mild to moderate hypertension[4]

In people with hypertension, how much reduction of blood pressure can be achieved with a low salt diet and how difficult is this to organise (and persist with)?

Whether our usual salt intake is a cause of hypertension or not, elevated blood pressure can usually be lowered by salt restriction. Diuretic drugs work by increasing urinary sodium excretion. Alternatively a sufficient reduction of dietary sodium can achieve the same degree of negative sodium balance. In mild to moderate hypertension, reduction of sodium intake (which can be monitored with 24 hour urinary sodium) to around 50 mmol/day will usually give a useful reduction of blood pressure so that the patient may be able to come off hypotensive drugs (or not start them) or reduce the dose (and with this the probability of side effects). Salt restriction increases sensitivity to all hypotensive drugs except slow channel calcium blockers, like nifedipine. Older people may be more responsive to salt reduction and they are particularly susceptible to side effects of drugs. Some people are more responsive than others. It has been reported that people with haptoglobin 1-1 genes are more likely to be sensitive to salt than those with haptoglobin 2-2.

Average percentages of sodium from different sources[5]

Discretionary	
Added at table	9·0
Used in cooking	6·0
Food	
Naturally occurring	18·5
Added salt in processing	58·7
Non-salt additives	7·2
Salt in water supply (average)	0·6
	100·0

Sodium in foods

High sodium (10 mmol or more per usual serving)

Ham, bacon, tongue, corned beef, salami, sausage, smoked fish. Most breakfast cereals. Baking powder, pickles, tomato sauce, tomato juice, soy sauce, anchovy paste. Most biscuits. Most cheeses, especially blue vein. Marmite, Bovril, olives. Canned vegetables, soups, pizzas, potato crisps.

Medium sodium:

Bread, cakes, milk, butter margarine, low salt cheeses (eg ricotta). Some mineral waters (eg Vichy).

Low sodium (1 mmol or less per usual serving)

Rice, oatmeal, plain (wheat) flour, most pasta. Coffee, tea, human milk. Fresh, canned, and dried fruit. Fresh and frozen vegetables. Potatoes. Fresh meat and poultry, fresh fish. Herbs and spices. Alcoholic drinks. Pepper, vinegar. Cream. Unprocessed bran. Matzos. Salt free products (bread, butter, margarine, breakfast cereals). Some mineral waters (eg Evian, Perrier, Vittel).

Body weight

People who don't eat enough food energy and lose weight usually have a fall of (normal) blood pressure.

If hypertensive obese patients reduce their weight they show falls of blood pressure like 10 mm systolic/5 mm diastolic for 5 kg weight loss.

Less food means less sodium eaten. Some weight loss occurs even if sodium intake is maintained, but the combination of weight loss and a low sodium intake is more effective.

In a randomised placebo controlled trial of first line treatment of mild hypertension in overweight patients, the weight reduction group (mean loss 7·4 kg) had a 13 mm Hg fall of systolic blood pressure while those treated with metoprolol (200 mg/d) had a 10 mm Hg fall. Plasma lipids improved in the weight reduction group, but changed adversely in those on drug therapy.[6]

Obese people are likely to have a higher blood pressure than lean people.

In a birth cohort of over 5000 people born in Britain in the same week, blood pressures at the age of 36 were progressively higher in those with a body mass index (weight (kg)/height (cm)^2) above 26.

Typically a 3 mm Hg higher diastolic pressure may be expected for every 10 kg increase in body weight. In a large Swedish study of 60 year old men, a quarter of the fattest fifth were taking antihypertensive drugs compared with only 4% of the thinnest fifth.[7]

Raised blood pressure and hyperlipidaemia are both major risk factors for cardiovascular disease, and effective weight reduction will improve both.

Diet and hypertension

Alcohol

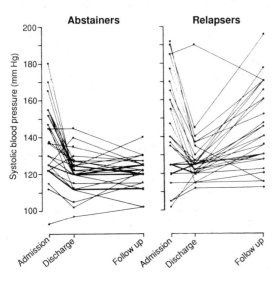

Alcohol intake is emerging as one of the important environmental factors associated with raised blood pressure. Heavy drinkers have higher blood pressure than light drinkers and abstainers. The effect starts above about three (stated) drinks a day. Systolic pressure is more affected than diastolic.

The pressor effect of alcohol can be demonstrated directly. It was seen, for example, in men with essential hypertension who were moderate to heavy drinkers. They continued their habitual intake of beer and antihypertensive drugs. When low alcohol beer (0·9% alcohol) was substituted for the same intake of regular beer (5% alcohol) blood pressure fell 5/3 mm Hg.[9]

The mechanism(s) have not yet been worked out. Acute ingestion of alcohol causes peripheral vasodilatation, but there are features of a hyperadrenergic state in the withdrawal syndrome. Plasma cortisol concentrations are sometimes raised in alcoholics. Increased red cell volume and hence increased blood viscosity is a possible mechanism.

When alcoholic patients were admitted to hospital for detoxification their systolic blood pressure fell by about 20 mm Hg; it stayed down if they continued to abstain, but rose again if alcohol drinking was resumed. The same pattern was seen with the diastolic pressure.[8]

Components in the diet that may lower blood pressure

Healthy (normotensive) hospital staff in Perth, Western Australia, were provided with all their meals as one of two diets—mixed omnivore or (lacto-ovo) vegetarian. Sodium intakes were kept the same.

After 6 weeks the subjects were switched to the other diet. Blood pressures were significantly lower by about 6 mm/3·5 mm Hg on the vegetarian diet.

Potassium in foods

Moderate to high (mmol per usual serving):

Potatoes (17), pulses (9-22), instant coffee (10), dried fruits (5-24), treacle (9), fresh meat and fish (8-10), All Bran (8), tomatoes, fresh fruit (2-10), beer (3-8), cows' milk (5), oatmeal (5), orange juice (4), nuts (2-6), wines (2-4), vegetables (1-7).

Low (1-3 mmol per usual serving):

Rice, chocolate, human milk, egg, biscuits, bread, cheese, flour, cornflakes.

Very low or absent:

Sugar, jam, honey, butter, margarine, cream, oils, spirits.

Potassium is the major intracellular cation; the more concentrated the cells in a food, the higher the potassium concentration.

The Ministry of Agriculture, Fisheries, and Food estimated that root vegetables provide a quarter of normal British people's intake, with fruit and other vegetables each providing 10% or less.

Potassium—In a placebo controlled crossover trial of mild to moderate hypertension, blood pressure fell by (average) 7/4 mm Hg with a supplement of eight Slow-K tablets (64 mmol potassium) a day. But the same (London) clinic found little or no effect in similar hypertensive patients who had managed to reduce their sodium intake (and urinary sodium) to around 70 mmol a day—that is, potassium acts as a sodium antagonist and has little effect when sodium intake has been halved.[10]

Potassium should be in the form of food. With pharmaceutical potassium there is concern that the risk of hyperkalaemia may be greater than the benefit of a small hypotensive effect.[11] (Pharmaceutical potassium, separately or incorporated in the diuretic tablet, may nevertheless be indicated for patients taking diuretics long term).

Magnesium—Magnesium can sometimes lower blood pressure. In patients who had received long term diuretics (mostly for hypertension) and potassium supplements half were also given magnesium aspartate hydrochloride for six months. Their blood pressure fell significantly. The diuretics had presumably led to subclinical magnesium depletion.

Magnesium is distributed in foods somewhat similarly to potassium. Bran, wholegrain cereals, and legumes are the richest sources. Most vegetables contain similar moderate amounts to meat.

1 Truswell AS, Kennelly BM, Hansen JDL, Lee RB. Blood pressures of !Kung Bushmen in northern Botswana. *Am Heart J* 1972;**84**:5–12.
2 Dahl LK. Salt and hypertension. *American Journal of Clinical Nutrition*, 1972;**25**:231–44.
3 Department of Health and Social Security. *Diet and Cardiovascular Disease*. London: HMSO, 1984. (Reports on Health and Social Subjects, No 28.)
4 Beard TC, Cooke HM, Gray WR, Barge R. Randomised controlled trial of a no-added-sodium diet for mild hypertension. *Lancet* 1982; ii: 455–8.
5 Edwards DG, Kaye AE, Druce E. Sources and intakes of sodium in the United Kingdom diet. *European Journal of Clinical Nutrition*, 1989;**43**:855–61.
6 McMahon SW, Macdonald GJ, Bernstein L, Andrews G, Blacket RB. Comparison of weight reduction with metoprolol in treatment of hypertension in young overweight patients. *Lancet* 1985;i:1233–5.
7 Larsson B, Björntorp P, Tibblin G. The health consequences of moderate obesity. *Int J Obes* 1981;**5**:97–116.
8 Saunders JB, Beevers DG, Paton A. Alcohol-induced hypertension. *Lancet* 1981;ii:653–6.
9 Puddey IB, Beilin LJ, Vandongen R. Regular alcohol use raises blood pressure in treated hypertensive subjects. *Lancet* 1987;i:647–50.
10 Smith SJ, Markandu MD, Sagnella GA, MacGregor GA. Moderate potassium chloride supplementation in essential hypertension: is it additive to moderate sodium restriction? *BMJ* 1985;**290**:110–3.
11 Anonymous. Fending off the potassium pushers. Editorial. *N Engl J Med* 1985;**312**:785–7.
12 Kestin M, Clifton P, Belling GB, *et al*. n-3 Fatty acids of marine origin lower systolic blood pressure and triglycerides but raise LDL cholesterol compared with n-3 and n-6 fatty acids from plants. *Am J Clin Nutr* 1990;**51**:1028–34.
13 Stamler R, Stamler J, Grimm R, *et al*. Nutritional therapy for high blood pressure. Final report of a 4-year randomized controlled trial. *JAMA* 1987;**257**:1484–91.

Polyunsaturated fatty acids—In earlier studies it appeared that blood pressure was sometimes lower when people changed from a Western diet to a "prudent", cholesterol lowering diet, with its decreased total fat and saturated fat and increased proportion of omega-6 polyunsaturated fat. But in several strictly controlled trials, in which only the type of fat or oil supplement was changed, there was a significant fall in blood pressure with fish body oil containing long chain omega-3 fatty acids but not with omega-6 polyunsaturated oils (such as corn or safflower oil).[12] The "dose" of omega-3 fatty acids was larger than could normally be obtained from eating more fish.

Calcium—Analyses of a diet and health survey in the United States suggested that people with low calcium intakes had more hypertension, and in Britain there is less cardiovascular disease in areas with hard water (which contains more calcium). Controlled trials with calcium supplements—usually 1·0 to 1·5 g/day—have shown late and small average reductions of blood pressure, and some trials have shown no effect. The benefit/cost is probably too small for calcium to be clinically useful as treatment for hypertension, but a small reduction in blood pressure could be a bonus when increased dietary calcium or calcium supplements are used to prevent postmenopausal osteoporosis.

Conclusion

Small rises in blood pressure are very commonly found in practice. Doctors may well hesitate to start prescribing hypotensive drugs, even if the high reading persists at the next visit. The combination of substantially reducing salt intake and body weight and limiting (standard) alcoholic drinks to only one or two a day is well worth a serious try in this circumstance,[13] and is likely to succeed if the patient is able to comply with all three sets of dietary advice.

3: NUTRITIONAL ADVICE FOR OTHER CHRONIC DISEASES

Dental caries

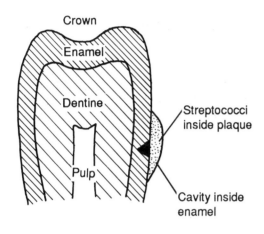

Dental caries affects people predominantly in the first 25 years of life. Dental enamel is the hardest material in the body. Its weakness is that, because it is basically calcium phosphate, it is dissolved by acid. Three factors together contribute to caries.

Infection—A specific species of viridans streptococci, *Streptococcus mutans*, metabolises sugars to lactic acid and polymerises sugars to a layer of covering polysaccharide in which the bacteria are shielded from saliva and the tongue. Some people harbour more of these bacteria than others.

Substrate—Most sugars serve as substrate—sucrose, glucose, fructose, and lactose (apparently not sorbitol or xylitol). Starches too, if they stay in the mouth are split to sugars by salivary amylase. Consumption of sugary foods between meals, especially if they are sticky and consumption is repeated, favours the development of caries. Brushing the teeth and flossing between them after meals reduces the likelihood of caries.

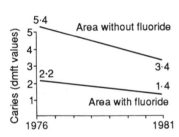

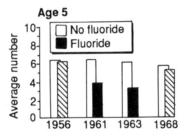

Resistance of the teeth—Caries is more likely in fissures. In older people the "mature" enamel is more resistant. An intake of 1–3 mg/day of fluoride—as occurs, for example, if drinking water is fluoridated at a concentration of 1 mg/l—increases the enamel's resistance, especially if taken while enamel is being laid down before the tooth erupts.

Fall in number of decayed, missing, filled teeth (dmft) at age 5 years in two areas, one with fluoridated water one without, between 1976 and 1981[1]

The shaded bars showed what happened to the number of decayed temporary teeth in Kilmarnock after fluoridation of water, which started in 1956 and was discontinued in 1962. Unshaded bars are findings in Ayr, which was never fluoridated[2]

Gall stones

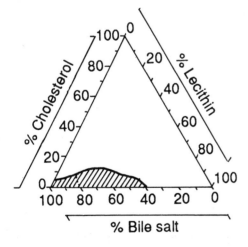

Three major components of bile (bile salts, lecithin, and cholesterol) on triangular coordinates. Each component is expressed as percentage moles of total bile salt, lecithin, and cholesterol. The shaded area shows conditions required for cholesterol to be soluble in micellar form. If the concentration of cholesterol goes up or bile acids or lecithin down then cholesterol is likely to precipitate out[3]

Most gall stones are composed mainly (about 85%) of crystallised cholesterol with small proportions of calcium carbonate, palmitate, and phosphate. Cholesterol, which is excreted by the liver into the bile, would be completely insoluble in an aqueous fluid like bile if it were not kept in micelle microemulsion by the combined detergent action of the bile acids and phospholipids (chiefly lecithin) in bile.

Non-dietary risk factors include female sex, pregnancy, oral contraceptives, age, ileal disease, surgery for peptic ulcer, clofibrate therapy, and certain ethnic groups—for example, Pima Amerindians have a high incidence of gall stones.

Dietary factors associated with this multifactorial condition are being worked out—for example, by the study of duodenal bile samples after cholecystokinin in people on different diets or by dietary histories in patients with gall stones compared with controls. They include: obesity; periods of fasting or missing meals; possibly high dietary cholesterol and high dietary sugar; low dietary fibre intake, especially wheat fibre; and total parenteral nutrition. A reported association with high intakes of polyunsaturated fat has not been confirmed, and no association has been found between gall stones and deviations of plasma cholesterol concentrations. Moderate alcohol intake appears to be protective.

These associations do not apply to the less common pigment stones.

Urinary tract stones

Foods rich in oxalate

Beetroots, cocoa, chocalate, currants, dried figs, rhubarb, parsley, spinach, tea, swiss chard, blackberries, gooseberries, oranges, strawberries, raspberries, turnip greens, carrots, green beans, onion, cucumbers, lemon peel.

Uric acid stones

One dietary cause of acid urine is a high protein intake. The amino acids methionine and cystine are metabolised to urinary sulphuric acid.

Food traditionally rich in purines include liver, kidneys, sweetbreads, sardines, anchovies, fish roes, and yeast extracts, but there are no modern tables and dietary RNA may raise plasma urate more than DNA.

Calcium stones—Dietary factors which tend to increase urinary calcium or have been associated with stones are high intakes of protein, sodium, refined carbohydrate, vitamin D, calcium (spread over the day), alcohol, curry, spicy foods, and Worcester sauce and low intakes of cereal fibre and water.

Oxalate stones—Associated dietary factors are high intakes of oxalate or vitamin C and low water intake.

Uric acid stones are associated with an acid urine, a high purine diet, and low water consumption.

The one common dietary association with all the common types of stone—and with the rare ones also—is a low water intake. Drinking plenty of water is an important habit for anyone liable to stones, especially if the weather is hot. Last thing at night is the important time to take it.

Diabetes mellitus

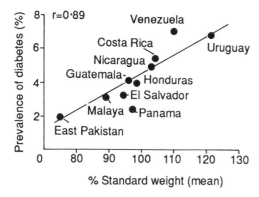

Relation of body weight to prevalence of diabetes (standardised criteria) between countries[4]

Development of insulin dependent (type I) diabetes is not related to antecedent diet. This type of diabetes occurs all over the world, and in undernourished communities it is the predominant type.

Non-insulin dependent (type II) diabetes, which is the more common type in affluent communities, is closely linked to obesity. It was observed as long ago as 400 BC in India that diabetes is a disease of the well fed in countries with food shortages. Death rates have fallen in each of the European wars in the last 120 years. The prevalence of diabetes is strongly correlated with indices of overweight both between countries and within countries.

Looked at another way, diabetes is the complication of obesity whose incidence goes up at the steepest gradient with degree of overweight. The risk of developing diabetes is greater in people whose obesity is mainly intra-abdominal rather than on the hips or buttocks (subcutaneous)—people with a high ratio of waist : hip circumferences.[6]

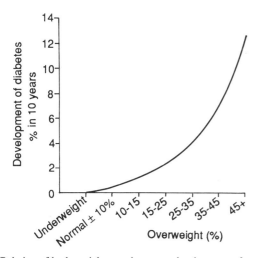

Relation of body weight to subsequent development of diabetes in 10 years[5]

Diabetes is, again, a multifactorial disease. There is a strong family influence, though this may be partly because eating habits and body weight are influenced by family behaviour. But a genetic factor is clear in some groups: the Pima Amerindians in North America and Micronesians in Nauru. When these people are obese (which most of them are these days) the incidence of diabetes (in older life) is over 50%.

Other chronic diseases

Diets and prevalence of diabetes* in 11 populations[4]

	Diabetes prevalence	Percentage of energy provided by:			
		Total carbohydrate	Sugar	Protein	Fat
East Pakistan	2·0	83	2	10	7
Panama	2·5	67	9	11	22
El Salvador	3·2	70	7	12	17
Malaya	3·3	68	8	11	21
Honduras	4·1	66	8	13	22
Guatemala	4·2	73	10	12	15
Nicaragua	5·0	66	12	13	21
Costa Rica	5·4	69	17	11	21
Uruguay	6·9	53	12	14	33
Venezuela	7·0	62	7	14	24
Bangor, Pa	17·2	47		13	40

* Venous blood glucose >8·3 mmol/l in patients aged over 30 years

The popular belief that eating a lot of *sugar* predisposes to diabetes is not confirmed by several epidemiological and prospective studies. High *fat* intake is more likely to lead to diabetes, a hypothesis first put forward in Britain in 1935 by Sir Harold Himsworth. High *total carbohydrate* (mostly starch) and high *fibre* intakes are characteristic of peasant communities, in which maturity onset diabetes is uncommon.

Chromium (in the organic compound, "glucose tolerance factor") appears to be necessary for the stimulation by insulin of glucose transport into cells, but chromium deficiency is a very rare cause of carbohydrate intolerance. This trace element must, however, be remembered in prolonged parenteral feeding.

Diets for managing established diabetes are discussed in chapter 13.

Cirrhosis of the liver

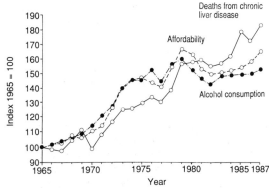

Alcohol affordability and consumption and deaths from cirrhosis in the UK, 1965–87. As alcohol became more affordable, consumption of alcohol and harm related to alcohol increased[8]

Countries with high alcohol consumption per head have high mortalities from cirrhosis. These have fallen when there has been a reduction in the supply of alcohol—for example, during prohibition in the USA and during the two world wars in Europe.

Correlation of alcohol consumption and deaths from cirrhosis between countries is close, but there are deviations. Britain has a lower incidence of cirrhosis than might be expected from the rate of alcohol consumption but mortality from cirrhosis has nearly doubled here in the last 25 years. Where alcohol consumption is high most cases of cirrhosis are due to alcohol. Other causes—for example, hepatitis B—account for about a third of cases in Britain.

Within countries the risk of developing cirrhosis is related to the dose and duration of alcohol intake. Daily heavy drinking for years is the typical pattern—80 g (eight drinks) a day in men, and usually well over this.

No precise safe level of alcohol intake can be given—only a clinical impression—because people who drink heavily underestimate their consumption when asked about it, and no prospective epidemiological study has been done. Women are more susceptible to hepatic damage from alcohol because they have smaller livers (where most metabolism of alcohol occurs) and also lower rates of gastric (first pass) oxidation of alcohol than men.[7] Not all heavy drinkers get cirrhosis; those with certain HLA antigens, such as B8 and B40, are more susceptible.

Although alcoholics may become deficient in nutrients, those who develop cirrhosis are often socially organised and well nourished. There is no evidence that a high protein diet or choline can prevent alcoholic cirrhosis in man. Even when cirrhosis is established, improved clinical state and prognosis may be expected in those who thereafter manage to abstain completely.

Some types of cancer

Oesophageal cancer

300 × range in incidence

Highest rates
   Linxian, People's Republic of China,
   East Mazandaran, Iran,
   and Transkei, South Africa

In Europe there are moderately high rates in NW France and in Switzerland

Differences in diets are thought to account for more variation in the incidence of all cancers than any other factor (with smoking in second order).[9] The big questions are which dietary components are active, and how do they work? Our bodies have three routes of entry for foreign compounds: the skin, lungs, and intestines. As a function of surface area the chances of absorption are skin 1, lungs 1000, and intestines 1 000 000. There are countless natural non-nutrient substances in foods and several are mutagens. The fact that they can induce mutations in a standard bacterial culture does not, however, establish that they are dangerous to man: there are many available protective mechanisms.

Diet may have a more decisive effect by weakening defence mechanisms than by supplying potent carcinogens. Epidemiologists estimate that synthetic chemical additives in food account for under 1% of all cancers.[9] The cancers most clearly related to habitual diet are oesophageal, gastric, and large intestinal cancers.

Oesophagus—In the Chinese focus of oesophageal cancer nitrosamines have been found in mouldy food and there is a deficiency of molybdenum. Domestic fowl are affected too. In the Iranian focus there are some vitamin deficiencies and people may take opium by mouth. In the Transkei researchers think that fusarium mycotoxins, together with deficiencies of niacin, zinc, and other micronutrients, are responsible for the new epidemic of oesophageal cancer. In Europe alcohol, especially that derived from apples, and tobacco are associated factors.

Stomach—Dietary factors associated with gastric cancer are the consumption of smoked salted fish, pickled foods, cured meats, and salt and lack of refrigeration. Foods that appear from surveys to be protective include salads and citrus fruit. A leading hypothesis is that nitrites in the stomach react with secondary amines and amides to produce nitrosamines and nitrosamides, some of which are potent carcinogens in animals. A small part of the nitrite comes from cured meats (bacon and ham). The nitrite keeps the colour pink and prevents botulism. But most swallowed nitrite is formed in the mouth by bacterial action on nitrates secreted in saliva. Our main source of nitrates is leafy and root vegetables. However, in Britain rates of gastric cancer are lower in regions (the south) where nitrate intake from vegetables and salivary nitrates are higher.[11] Perhaps the vegetables contain anticarcinogens such as ascorbic acid, which inhibits nitrosation. Refrigeration reduces secondary amine formation in foods rich in protein. When gastric acid output is low bacteria colonise the stomach and more nitrites are produced.

Large intestine[12]—Comparisons between countries and many of the case-control studies show that total fat intake and meat (or protein) intake are related to large bowel cancer. Fat and protein intakes are themselves correlated, and it is not yet clear which is the primary relation. One cause of intestinal cancer may be the highly mutagenic quinoline derivatives (IQ, MeIQ, MeIQx, etc) that are formed when foods rich in protein are cooked at high temperatures. Another possible cause is the larger than usual amounts of bile acid metabolites, which may be mutagenic, that may be found in the colonic lumens of people who eat high fat diets. Both wheat fibre and brassica vegetables appear to be protective. Most cancers of the large intestine arise in polyps. If malignant transformation in polyps can be delayed by diet this will be valuable public health information. Prevention trials are being undertaken at present in several centres, testing such interventions as increased wheat fibre or β carotene and decreased fat intake. Some types of beer have been associated with rectal cancer. There have, however, been variations and inconsistencies in all the case-control studies. Apart from diet, there is a familial influence; rectal cancer is commoner in men, and cholecystectomy increases the risk of cancer of the colon.

Gastric cancer

The incidence in Britain has spontaneously fallen to half in the past 25 years.

There have been similar reductions in many developed countries.[10]

Highest rates, in Japan, are 5 times those in England and Wales, 10 times those in the USA, 25 times those in parts of east Africa.

Chronic atrophic gastritis is a precancerous state.

Cancer of the large bowel

The second largest cause of death from cancer (after lung cancer in men and breast cancer in women).

It is 10 times more common in developed Western countries like Britain and USA than in the Third World.

Rates in Scotland have been among the highest in the world.

The epidemiology of rectal cancer shows some minor differences from the larger group of colon cancer.

1 French AD, Carmichael CL, Rugg-Gunn AJ, *et al*. Fluoridation and dental caries experience in 5 year old children in Newcastle and Northumberland in 1981. *Br Dent J* 1984;**156**:54–7.
2 Department of Health and Social Security. *The fluoridation studies in the United Kingdom and the results achieved after eleven years*. London: HMSO, 1969. (Reports on Public Health and Medical Subjects No 122.)
3 Small DM. Gallstones. *N Engl J Med* 1969;**279**:588–93.
4 West KM, Kalbfleisch JM. Influence of nutritional factors on prevalence of diabetes. *Diabetes* 1971;**20**:99–108.
5 Westlund K, Nicolayson R. Ten year mortality and morbidity related to serum cholesterol. *Scand J Clin Lab Invest* 1972;**30**:3–24.
6 Ohlson LO, Larsson B, Svarsudd K, *et al*. The influence of body fat distribution on the incidence of diabetes mellitus. 13·5 years of follow up of the participants in the study of men born in 1913. *Diabetes* 1985;**34**:1055–8.
7 Frezza M, di Padova C, Pozzato G. High blood alcohol levels in women. The role of decreased gastric alcohol dehydrogenase activity and first-pass metabolism. *N Engl J Med* 1990;**322**:95–9.
8 Department of Health. *On the state of the public health for the year 1988*. London: HMSO, 1989;fig 2.1.
9 Doll R, Peto R. The causes of cancer: qualitative estimates of avoidable risks of cancer in the United States today. *JNCI* 1981;**66**:1191–308.
10 Howson CP, Hiyama T, Wynder EL. The decline in gastric cancer: epidemiology of an unplanned triumph. *Epidemiol Rev* 1986;**8**:1–27.
11 Forman D, Al-Dabbagh S, Doll R. Nitrates, nitrites and gastric cancer in Great Britain. *Nature* 1985;**313**:620–5.
12 Cummings JH, Bingham SA. Dietary fibre, fermentation and large bowel cancer. *Cancer Surveys* 1987;**6**:601–21.

4: NUTRITION FOR PREGNANCY

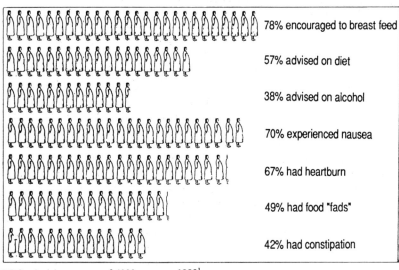

78% encouraged to breast feed

57% advised on diet

38% advised on alcohol

70% experienced nausea

67% had heartburn

49% had food "fads"

42% had constipation

BBC television survey of 6000 women, 1982[1]

Pregnancy is a time when appetite is altered and nutritional needs change. What the expectant mother eats or drinks can affect her baby's health and her own comfort. In pregnancy women develop a new interest in the consequences for health of what they eat. They are entitled to advice from their doctors.

Nutrition for pregnancy

Women who had had a baby with a neural tube defect and intended becoming pregnant again were entered into a multicentre trial coordinated by R W Swithells.[2] Only 3/387 women taking a periconceptional supplement of eight vitamins, iron, and calcium subsequently had babies with neural tube defects compared with a 6·5 times higher rate in unsupplemented women.

This was not a randomised or blind trial,[3] so from 1983 to 1991 the MRC conducted a randomised, double blind trial in seven countries comparing four supplements taken periconceptionally by 1195 women. With folic acid (0·4 mg) there were 0·7% neural tube defects, only one fifth (significant) the rate with the other nutritional supplements.[4]

Pregnant women who subsequently have babies with neural tube defects tend to have somewhat low red cell folates but not in the "deficient" range. Folate is needed for DNA synthesis and it seems that an adequate supply is especially critical in the embryo at the time the neural tube closes.

Before pregnancy the first advice should ideally be communicated when a woman decides to try to have a baby. Pregnancies in women who are overweight, have anorexia nervosa, or whose growth is not completed are more difficult, and these women need extra nutritional care.

A good intake of folate may be important in preventing neural tube defects in a minority of women. If so the stage when this vitamin is needed is around 28 days after ovulation—that is, supplementation has to be periconceptional. Likewise, it is the early weeks when excess alcohol intake may lead to malformations.

During pregnancy extra nutrients are required, especially from 20 weeks, for the fetus and for the placenta. Tissue is also laid down in the uterus and breasts, blood volume is increased, and, in healthy women with adequate food, adipose tissue increases by around 2·7 kg. This fat is deposited mostly on the hips and thighs.

Alcohol in pregnancy[5][6]

Heavy drinkers have a greatly increased risk of inducing the fetal alcohol syndrome—characteristic underdevelopment of the mid face, small size, and mental retardation.

Women who intend to become pregnant should not sit drinking whatever the occasion: they could be two or three weeks pregnant.

Once pregnancy is established the rule should be no more than one alcoholic drink a day to be sure of preventing minor effects, chiefly growth retardation.

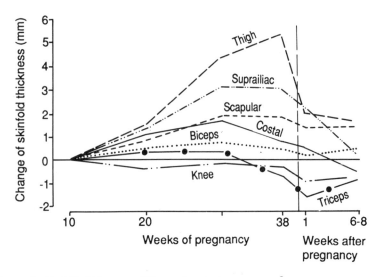

Changes in skinfold thickness at different sites during pregnancy[7]

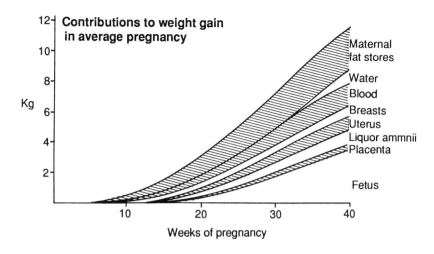

Contributions to weight gain in average pregnancy

The need for extra energy for pregnancy works out to about 250 MJ (60 000 kcal).[8] This includes storage in fetal fat and protein and in maternal reproductive tissues and adipose tissue and takes account of the mother's increased basal metabolic rate and the energy needed to move a heavier body. This corresponds to 1 MJ (240 kcal) a day (excluding the first month, for 250 days), and in Britain the recommended daily intake of energy during pregnancy (10 MJ, 2400 kcal) until 1991* was 1 MJ (240 kcal) above the non-pregnant amount (9 MJ or 2150 kcal). When actual food intakes are carefully measured, however, little indication exists of extra energy intake in Western women. This has been found in recent careful intake measurements in London, Cambridge, Aberdeen, Glasgow, Wageningen, and Sydney. In all these centres women were found to eat an average of almost 9 MJ (2150 kcal). Pregnant women seem to reduce their exercise if they can. Their energy metabolism may also become more efficient. Postprandial cholecystokinin concentrations increase, which enhances nutrient absorption and the anabolic actions of insulin.

The amounts of different nutrients which the mother has to put into her fetus by the time of delivery have been worked out by chemical analysis of stillbirths. These can be estimated more accurately for stable inorganic elements than for the vitamins. From these figures for nutrients accumulated and from information on whether there is any change in their turnover the extra requirements for pregnancy can be estimated.

The metabolism of protein is more efficient and so is absorption of iron in pregnancy.

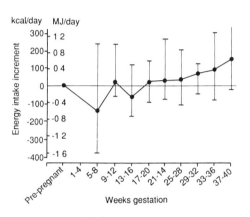

Energy intake increments (and confidence limits) for 71 women throughout pregnancy[9]

For most nutrients like *protein* the small extra amounts required are covered adequately by a normal diet. But intakes are more critical for the other five nutrients in the table showing recommended daily intakes.

Folate is the only vitamin and calcium the only nutrient element whose requirement doubles in pregnancy. Serum and red cell folate concentrations decline in pregnancy and, if looked for, some degree of megaloblastic change can be found in substantial minorities of women in late pregnancy. Such changes have been reported in 6-25% of women not taking supplements in Britain. The word folate comes from the Latin *folia* (leaf) because it was first found in spinach, but food sources are not the same as for vitamin C. Liver and kidneys, whole grain cereals, nuts, and legumes are good sources of folate, whereas fruits are fairly poor (about 5 μg/100 g). The folate content of vegetables varies from about 10 μg/100 g in potatoes and carrots up to 300 μg in endive; the vitamin is largely destroyed by prolonged boiling.

With *calcium*, absorption is likely to become more efficient. Without any change of vitamin D intake or exposure to the sun plasma concentrations of calcitriol (the active form of the vitamin converted in the kidney) are increased. The easiest way of obtaining the extra calcium needed for pregnancy and lactation is from milk; ½ litre supplies about 600 mg calcium (as does 60 g Cheddar cheese).

Recommended daily intakes* for six critical nutrients in pregnancy[10]

	Addition for pregnancy	Non-pregnant women	Total
Protein (g)	+10	50	60
Folate (μg total folate)	+220	180	400
Calcium (mg)	+400	800	1200
Iron (mg)	+15	15	30
Zinc (mg)	+3	12	15
Iodine (μg)	+25	150	175

* United States recommended dietary allowances, 1989

Good sources of folate (total folate, μg/100 g)

About 250 μg: liver, bran, endive (Marmite, Bovril, and yeast contain about 1000 μg/100 mg, but servings are very small)

About 100 μg: broccoli tops, spinach, Brussels sprouts, nuts, kidneys, peas, All Bran

About 50 μg: oatmeal, avocado, boiled beetroot, egg yolk, wholemeal bread, peanut butter, oranges

Legumes contain over 100 μg raw, but this is usually reduced to about a fifth after cooking.

---

* In 1991 the DoH revised the estimated average extra requirement of energy in pregnancy to 0·8 MJ (200 kcal) a day.

Nutrition for pregnancy

The *iron* contents of the fetus (about 300 mg), placenta (50 mg), and average postpartum blood loss (200 mg) add up to some 550 mg. The red cell mass also increases after 12 weeks by an amount which corresponds to about another 500 mg of iron, but this is a temporary internal borrowing from stores and causes no extra demand provided the stores are sufficient. Against these extra needs there is the saving from no menstruation (some 200 mg) and improved intestinal absorption.

Maternal haemoglobin concentration declines by about 10% because of physiological haemodilution; and serum iron concentration, transferrin saturation, and ferritin concentration all go down. These changes can be partly—but only partly—prevented by iron supplementation.

The plasma *zinc* concentration falls by about 30% in pregnancy, and this is apparently not prevented by zinc supplementation. Many pregnant women are found to eat less than the current recommended dietary intakes. The zinc concentration in cord blood is usually about double that in the puerperal mother's blood. There is, of course, haemodilution in pregnancy and the plasma zinc concentration falls when oral contraceptives are taken so these observations do not prove deficiency. But white cell zinc concentration falls in pregnancy too (this correlates with muscle zinc), and white cell zinc was significantly lower in mothers who had small for dates babies in a London study. More research is still needed, but in the meantime foods rich in zinc should be recommended as they are also good sources of other nutrients.

The increased need for *iodine* may be taken for granted in Britain, but in areas where goitre is endemic there is a risk of cretinism so expectant mothers should be given an injection of iodised oil, preferably before conception.

Weight gain

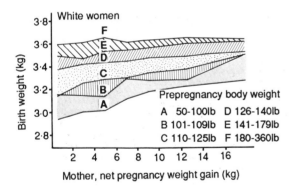

Birthweight is related positively to amount of maternal weight gain and to pre-pregnancy weight of the mother[11]

The amount of weight gained from before conception to shortly before delivery ranges considerably in normal women—from about 6 to 24 kg. A good average to try and keep close to is 12 kg (26 lb). This might be made up by about 115 g ($\frac{1}{4}$ lb)/week for the first 10 weeks and 300 g ($\frac{2}{3}$ lb)/week for the remaining 30 weeks. A mother's height, her weight for height at the start of pregnancy, and her weight gain can all influence the size of her fetus. Birth weights are lower in babies of mothers who choose (against medical advice) to continue to smoke during pregnancy.

In Third World countries, where mothers often start small and thin and gain little weight because of restricted and bulky food and heavy physical work, birthweights are lower than in affluent communities. They have been increased by providing food (energy) supplements during pregnancy in controlled trials. Average gains of birthweight in eight different trials have been 40 to 300 g.

Obesity in pregnancy increases the chances of a heavier and fatter baby and also of hypertension and gestational diabetes. Since 3 to 4 kg of the usual 12 kg weight gain is fat, obese women should try to put on only 7 to 8 kg overall during their pregnancy.

Hypertension and "toxaemia"

In pregnancy-induced hypertension (toxaemia) no excess of sodium is retained. It is proportional to the fluid retained.

No evidence exists that either a high or a low salt diet predisposes to pregnancy-induced hypertension or that any other dietary component—energy, protein, or any micronutrient—is directly responsible.

Diet and discomforts of pregnancy

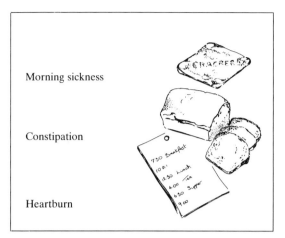

Morning sickness

Constipation

Heartburn

| **Vegans** | Must take vitamin B-12 supplements |
| **Other vegetarians** | May need to improve their intakes of iron and protein—for example by eating plenty of legumes and nuts |

Morning sickness is not always experienced in the morning. Some women have it in the evenings. There has been no controlled trial of simple management. One opinion is that it is related to a low blood glucose concentration and that a dry biscuit or similar light snack before getting up may help. It now seems possible that the increased cholecystokinin concentration could explain the symptoms. Unlike other conditions that cause nausea, women tend to put on weight during the phase of morning sickness.[13]

Constipation and its complication haemorrhoids are very common in pregnancy. All pregnant women should be advised to eat more wholemeal bread, bran, or bran cereals to loosen and increase the bulk of their faeces.

Heartburn should improve if the woman eats smaller meals and avoids foods which she finds indigestible. The common meal pattern of tiny breakfast, small lunch, and large dinner becomes unsuitable in late pregnancy. It is a good plan for her to have four, five, or even six small meals throughout the day.

Cravings and aversions—At some stage in pregnancy most women experience a distortion of their usual range of likes and dislikes of foods. Women may develop a nine month aversion to foods they usually like—for example, fried foods, coffee, tea. Contrariwise and at the same time they may experience a craving for certain foods. These are often sweet foods, such as fruits and chocolate ice cream, and sometimes salty, but some remarkable non-foods—coal, soap, soil—have been recorded.

Vegetarians who are pregnant may need extra dietary advice. There are several types of vegetarian (see chapter 7). Those most at risk are vegans. It is essential for them to take a supplement of vitamin B-12 for normal cerebral development of the fetus. Other lacto-ovo vegetarians, especially if they are prosperous and belong to a traditional vegetarian group, usually manage well enough but may want or need advice to optimise their protein and iron intakes. Legumes and nuts are an important part of a balanced vegetarian diet.

1 Boyd C, Sellers L. *The British way of birth*. London: Pan, 1982.
2 Swithells RW, Sheppard S, Wild J, Schorah CJ. Prevention of neural tube defect recurrences in Yorkshire: final report. *Lancet* 1989;ii:498–9
3 Wald NJ, Polani PE. Neural tube defects and vitamins: the need for a randomised clinical trial. *Br J Obstet Gynaecol* 1984;**91**:516–23.
4 MRC Vitamin Study Research Group. Prevention of neural tube defects: results of Medical Research Council vitamin study. *Lancet* 1991;**338**:131–7.
5 Beattie JO, Day RE, Cockburn F, Garg RA. Alcohol and the fetus in the West of Scotland. *BMJ* 1983;**287**:17–20.
   (Fetal alcohol syndrome in 40 heavy drinkers)
6 Sulaiman ND, Florey C du V, Taylor DJ, Ogston SA. Alcohol consumption in Dundee primigravidas and its effects on outcome of pregnancy. *BMJ* 1988;**296**:1500–3.
   (Well designed cohort study)

7 Taggart NR, Holliday RM, Billewicz WZ, Hytten FE, Thomson AM. Changes in skinfolds during pregnancy. *Br J Nutr* 1967;**21**:439–51.
8 Durnin JVGA. Energy requirements of pregnancy: an integration of the longitudinal data from the five country study. *Lancet* 1987;ii:1131–3.
9 Durnin JVGA, McKillop FM, Grant S, Fitzgerald G. Energy requirements of pregnancy in Scotland. *Lancet* 1987;ii:897–900.
10 Subcommittee on the 10th edition of the recommended dietary allowances, Food and Nutrition Board, National Research Council. *Recommended dietary allowances*. 10th ed. Washington DC: National Academy Press, 1989.
11 Naeye RL. In: Dobbing J, ed. *Maternal nutrition: eating for two?* London: Academic Press, 1981.
12 Report of a Study Group. *The hypertensive disorders of pregnancy*. Geneva: World Health Organisation, 1989. (Technical Report Series No 758.)
13 Uvnäs-Moberg K. The gastrointestinal tract in growth and reproduction. *Scientific American* 1989; July:60–5.

5: INFANT FEEDING

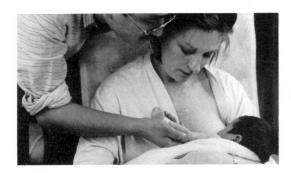

Infant feeding is the dominant nutritional interest in Third World countries and it gets much attention in Western countries because infants depend on others to feed them. For their first few months babies are fed only one food, so its composition is much more critical than the compositions of the many different foods in a mixed diet. Babies cannot eat ordinary adult food or say how they feel after the feed. Though there are still many questions, scientific knowledge is probably fuller about nutrition for this age of man than any other.

Breast or bottle?

Advantages of breast feeding

- Breast milk is microbiologically clean

- Breast feeding is natural and may confer benefits that science doesn't yet know about

- It provides anti-infective components: lymphocytes, macrophages, immunoglobulins (especially IgA), lactoferrin, lysozyme, complement, oligosaccharides (bifidus factor), growth factors, and modulators

- Many of the differences in composition between cows' and human milk have been minimised in modern infant formulas, but by no means all, and some nutrients such as iron and zinc are known to be better absorbed from human milk by babies

- For most women breast feeding is a satisfying, convenient, and enjoyable experience that is beneficial to the mother–child relationship

- Allergic reactions are less likely

- Mothers' milk is always at the right temperature

- A mother can always change from breast to bottle feeding but not the other way

For the first 4 to 6 months of life the infant should be fed either by breast feeding or on a formula based on cows' milk modified to make its composition suitable for infants—that is, more like breast milk. The decision which method to start with should be made well before delivery, and it should be made by the mother. The doctor's role is to give advice to help her make up her mind and then, whichever method she wants to use, to provide support and arrange instruction.

Breast feeding is recommended by the Department of Health and all authorities; the organisation of maternity wards, control of advertising, and change of social attitudes all make it easier than it used to be. On the other hand, modern technology makes bottle feeding easy and safe and the newer infant formulas are closer to breast milk in composition.

"Breastfeeding from a woman who is in good health and nutritional status provides a complete food, which is unique to the species. There is no better nutrition for healthy infants at term and during the early months of life . . . Breast feeding is preferable to feeding with infant formulas and should be encouraged."

DHSS
Present Day Practice in Infant Feeding (3rd report), 1988[1]

Composition of cows' milk compared with human milk and a modified infant formula (breast milk substitute). (All per 100 ml)

	Human* (mature)[2][3]	Cows' (full cream) (unfortified)	A modified milk formula† (powder diluted as directed
Energy (kcal)	70	67	69
Protein (total) (g)	1·1	3·5	1·5
Casein (% protein)	40%	80%	40%
Carbohydrate (g)	7·4	5·0	7·2
Fat (total) (g)	4·2	3·7	3·6
Saturated fat (% fat)	46%	66%	44%
Linoleic (% fat)	7–11%	3%	17%
Sodium (mmol)	0·6	2·2	0·71
Calcium (mg)	35	120	49
Phosphorus (mg)	15	95	30
Iron (mg)	0·075	0·050	0·9
Vitamin C (mg)	3·8	1·5	6·9
Vitamin D (µg)	0·8	0·15	1·1

* The composition of breast milk varies considerably with stage of lactation, between individuals, and with maternal nutrition.
† Mean of Cow and Gate Premium and SMA-S26.

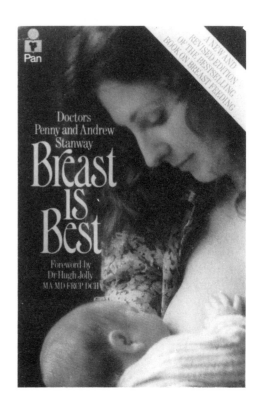

In Third World countries breast feeding unquestionably reduces infant mortality.

In affluent countries, however, epidemiologists have difficulty in showing an appreciable reduction in mortality when other factors are taken into account. Mothers who breast feed tend to have higher educational and income levels. A well designed study in Dundee seems to have corrected for all such confounding variables. It showed that breast feeding for the first 3 months of life confers a protection against gastrointestinal illness, which persists beyond the period of breast feeding itself.[4]

Prevalence of breast feeding in Great Britain, 1985[5] (For comparison the prevalence of breast feeding in Australia in 1983 was 85% on discharge from hospital and 54% at 3 months.[6])

How to manage breast feeding

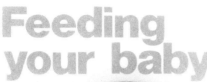

A BRITISH MEDICAL ASSOCIATION PUBLICATION

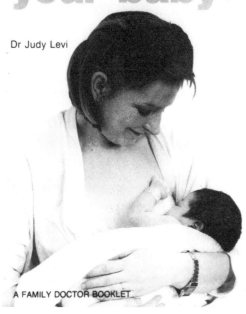

Feeding your baby

Dr Judy Levi

A FAMILY DOCTOR BOOKLET

Other publications and help obtainable from:

National Childbirth Trust
Breastfeeding Promotion Group
Alexandra House
Oldham Terrace
Acton
London W3 6NH

La Leche League
PO Box BM 3424
London WC1V 6XX

Association of Breastfeeding Mothers
7 Maybourne Close
Springfield Road
London SW26 6HQ

Knowing how to establish breast feeding is no longer instinctive in the women of our complex industrial societies. Some take to it naturally but others will not do well without guidance and a sympathetic environment.

• The mother should be adequately nourished during pregnancy.

• She should have watched others breast feeding and talked about it.

• She needs to involve and consider her husband. There can be sexual implications in breast feeding. His support (or opposition) will be important.

• The National Childbirth Trust or La Leche League can help to provide instruction and information.

• The baby should be put to the breast as soon as possible after delivery.

• The midwife can play an important part, giving advice on positioning the baby and encouragement in the first few days.[7]

• Frequent suckling stimulates prolactin secretion. Suckling more than six times a day maintains high basal prolactin as well as initiating prolactin surges with feeding.

• Feeding should be on demand or baby led.

• After delivery the baby should be in a crib next to its mother all or most of the time and suckled whenever it seems to be hungry. Colostrum is a valuable anti-infective fluid.

• Relaxation and privacy are needed.

• The baby should not be given other complementary milk—only water if necessary.

• The baby should feed from both breasts each time and start the feed with the breast used last.

• Advice may be needed about sore nipples or breasts, oversupply, or undersupply.

A one hour video for parents entitled *Breastfeeding—if you want to you can* (1988) (cost £9·99) is obtainable from Family Circle Magazine and other video outlets or from Pendulum Communications, PO Box 180, Beckenham, Kent BR3 2YJ

Infant feeding

Nutrition for the lactating mother

Except in malnourished communities, there is little evidence that dietary calories, protein, fat, water, or anything else have a consistent effect on milk volume. Regular and fairly frequent suckling is the well established stimulus. Human lactation works more by pull than by push.

Some constituents in the milk are affected by the mother's intake. (1) Fatty acid pattern, vitamin A, thiamin, riboflavin, biotin, folate, vitamin B-12, and vitamin C are affected, especially downwards if the mother's diet is deficient. (2) Zinc, iron, fluoride, and vitamin D may be responsive in some circumstances, but more research is needed. (3) Protein, lactose, fat content, calcium—that is, the major proximate constituents of milk—do not appear to be affected. (4) Specific proteins in the mother's diet might be excreted intact in small amounts and an allergic (IgE) reaction occasionally occurs in the baby. (5) The amount of caffeine in the milk after a cup of coffee is only about 1% of the maternal dose. Likewise, the alcohol concentration of breast milk is about the same as that of plasma. Single drinks of coffee or alcohol, well spaced out, are harmless, but the babies of alcoholics can be affected. Beer stimulates prolactin secretion (at least in non-lactating women) and so might increase lactation. Milk production is reduced in heavy smokers. (6) The fat-soluble environmental contaminants, polychlorinated biphenyls, dry cleaning solvents, and organochlorine insecticides (DDT, etc), are stored in adipose tissue and excreted in the cream of breast milk (though the DDT group is fairly innocuous in man). Lactating women should not go on to weight reducing diets, which might mobilise lipid contaminants from body fat so that they appear in the milk.

Extra nutrients needed by lactating compared with non-lactating women

Extra per day[8]	Percentage extra
About 850 ml water	
About 2·2 MJ	
(525 kcal) energy	24
16 g protein	36
45 mg vitamin C	150
150 µg folate	75
450 µg vitamin A	60
400 mg calcium	50
0·4 mg thiamin	50
6 mg zinc	50
50 µg iodine	42
10 µg vitamin D	*

* Non-pregnant adults do not normally require a dietary source of vitamin D unless they are housebound and deprived of exposure to sunlight

The mother's need for extra nutrients

A good average production of breast milk is 850 ml/day, and the mother's extra nutritional requirements are calculated from this and the average composition of milk (see table), taking into account the efficiency of absorption.

Most of the nutrients come along with the extra calories; lactating women usually have a good appetite and if this is satisfied by a mixed diet the nutrients that need watching (because there is little excess in the diets of non-lactating women) are calcium, iron, folate, and vitamin D. The extra calcium can come from a pint of milk or two cartons of yoghurt. Iron supplements may be advisable, and vitamin D supplements are recommended for any mother whose vitamin D status is in doubt (such as Asian mothers eating a wholly vegeterian diet). Folate deficiency incurred during pregnancy may first show as anaemia in the puerperium.

Ending lactation

In an industrial population the prevalence of breast feeding goes down with infant's age in a curve reminiscent of first order elimination kinetics. A few mothers continue breast feeding towards or beyond 12 months. In a British national sample the major reasons for stopping in the first 6 weeks were insufficient milk (54%) and painful breasts or painful or inverted nipples (18%); the commonest reason for stopping between 6 and 16 weeks was also insufficient milk (66%). Those with insufficient milk early never got lactation well established. Those with insufficient milk later may have had normal volume production but the baby started to outgrow this.

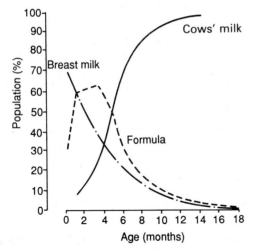

Mean consumption of different types of milk in normal Canadian infants.[9]

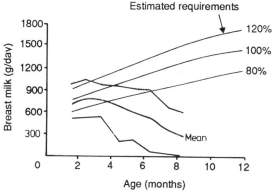

Measured breast milk intakes of Cambridge infants. Mean and ranges against estimated requirements.[10]

Complementary and supplementary bottles of milk

Complementary bottle feeds are used to finish off a breast feed and supplementary bottle feeds to replace a breast feed. The occasional bottle feed once a day or less is convenient if the mother has to leave the baby with a friend, but regular topping up of the baby's intake with bottle milk is likely to reduce sucking and breast milk production. Some mothers produce less milk than others, however, and if the baby is not gaining and hungry on pure breast feeding with good technique extra bottle feeding may be necessary.

Bottle feeding

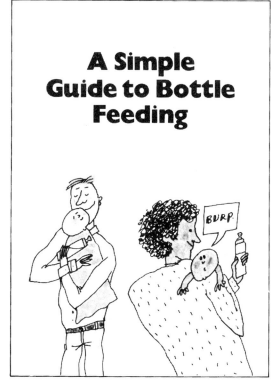

A booklet for parents from the Health Education Council.

Babies cannot cope with solid food in the first few months because:
● The extrusion reflex prevents spoon feeding
● They cannot swallow solids
● Pancreatic amylase is not adequately produced
● There is an increased likelihood of absorption of intact foreign (food) proteins
● Supplements may decrease iron absorption from breast milk and its anti-infection properties.

Some mothers choose to bottle feed from the start and others will change over from breast to bottle feeding after weeks or months, so they need practical advice.

● A cows' milk formula specially modified for infants should be used in which the protein has been reduced, the casein partly replaced by whey, the fat made more unsaturated, the lactose increased, sodium and calcium reduced, and enough of all the essential micronutrients added.

● Bottles and teats should be washed in water and detergent (the bottle brush used only for this) rinsed and sterilised by boiling in water or by standing covered in sterilising solution (usually hypochlorite) in a plastic container. It saves time to prepare several bottles at once. Empty the water out of each bottle, without touching the inside, then fill to the mark with recently boiled water that has cooled some minutes, not too hot or it will destroy some vitamins and may produce clumping.

● Exactly the amount of powder in the manufacturer's instructions should be put into the (wide mouthed) bottle, using the scoop provided (levelled with a clean knife, not pressed down). "One for the pot" can lead to obesity. Mothers and even nurses are often found to prepare feeds inaccurately. Screw on the cap and shake the bottle well. Bottles may be kept in the refrigerator for up to 24 hours.

● If the hole in the teat is too small it can lead to aerophagia or underfeeding. Milk should drip from the inverted teat at about 1 drop per second. Teats need replacing every few weeks.

● Babies do not mind cold milk but usually prefer it warm. The bottle should not be warmed for too long and the milk's temperature should be checked by dropping some on the parent's skin. Infant feed should not be warmed in a microwave oven once it is in the feeding bottle. Very hot fluid at the centre of the bottle may be missed and may scald the baby.[1] For about the first 8 weeks of life babies need to be fed every three to four hours, including the small hours of the morning. By the end of the first week most babies are taking 120–200 ml/kg per day (160 ml/kg corresponds to the old $2\frac{1}{2}$ fluid ounces per lb bodyweight).

● Cereals or rusks should not be added to milk in the bottle and babies should not be left to sleep with a bottle in their mouth.

● Vitamin drops, fruit juices, are not required as supplements to modern infant formulas.

● Uncles, grannies, and baby sitters can give a bottle feed but parents should feed their infant themselves as much as possible with the same sort of closeness, cuddling, and communication as in breast feeding.

Infant feeding

Weaning

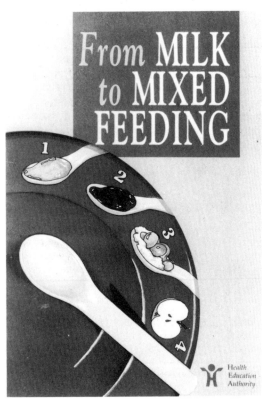

A booklet obtainable from the Health Education Authority.

Young infants cannot deal properly with solid foods (in reality semisolid foods at first) for the first 3 or 4 months. The natural time for starting solids (beikost) is when the energy provided by well established breast feeding starts to become insufficient. The Department of Health and other authorities advise that the introduction of any food to the baby, other than milk, should be unnecessary before the age of 3 months, but mothers may be tempted to jump the gun. Most babies should start a mixed diet not later than the age of 6 months.

Weight in the lower half of the standard percentiles without other symptoms is not an indication to augment breast feeding. Breast fed babies tend to put on weight (and length) a little more slowly than bottle fed infants. Indeed, the standard percentiles, derived mostly from bottle fed babies, may not be ideal. The time to start thinking about adding solids is when the infant still seems hungry after a good milk feed. But by 6 months stores of several nutrients, such as iron, zinc, and vitamin C, are often falling in exclusively milk fed infants, whether from breast or bottle.

When solids are introduced single ingredient foods should be used and started one at a time at half weekly intervals so that there is time to recognise allergy or other intolerance to each food. A little of the food on the tip of a teaspoon is enough at first, given after a milk feed when the baby is wide awake.

Infant cereals (usually enriched with iron) are traditional foods to start with; rice is better before wheat. They can be thinned with baby's usual milk (mother's or formula) or water. Thereafter different soft foods can be added: mashed potato; soft porridges; puréed fruit and vegetables, meat, or chicken. Foods should be semisolid—sieved or blended or commercial baby food. It is nutritionally sensible to give a balance of foods from the four major food groups: cereals, vegetables/fruit, dairy products, and meats/fish. Combination foods should not be given until tolerance to their individual components is established. Egg should not be started before 6 months because of the chance of allergic reactions, and then it is best to begin with a small amount of cooked yolk. Spinach, turnip, and beets can contain enough nitrate to cause methaemoglobinaemia in young infants. Coffee and tea should not be given. Babies should not be left alone while they are eating.

In the second 6 months other liquids can be given from a cup, especially citrus fruit juices. Untreated cows' milk can sometimes cause gastrointestinal bleeding from irritation by the bovine serum albumin. This does not happen with boiled milk or infant formulas (which have been heat treated). It is wrong to add any salt to the foods given to infants. A fully breast fed infant receives only about one thirtieth of the sodium in a typical British adult diet. There has been a quiet revolution in commercial baby foods; most contain no added salt or colours and only up to 4% sugar (with sour fruits). Infants' sodium intakes have been found to shoot up after 6 months but more from home prepared rather than commercial baby foods.

In the second 6 months

An increasing range of foods is given in the second 6 months. Variety is likely to cover the needs for most nutrients and provide a basis for healthy food habits. Some fruits or vegetables should be given each day, but the most critical nutrients at this stage are protein and iron: finely minced beef and legumes should be given regularly and the protein in cereal foods should not usually be diluted by refining or by added fat or sugar. Foods should become progressively more chewy and fibrous and include rusks and other finger foods like bread or cheese. Babies do not usually like strongly flavoured foods like pickled onions. Nuts, popcorn, raw peas, and similar small hard foods should be avoided; they can be breathed in accidentally. Commercial baby food manufacturers offer a succession of "strained", "junior", and "toddler" foods for maturing babies, and similar meals are usually made at home. Some cookbooks for babies are more sensible than others.

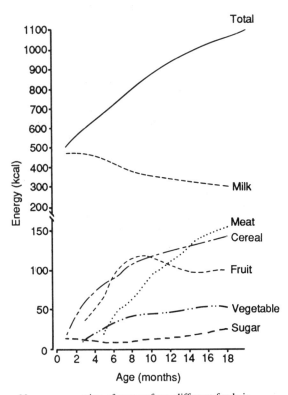

Mean consumption of energy from different foods in normal Canadian infants.[9]

A suggested timetable for introduction of solid foods:

1–4 months	Breast milk only
4–6 months	Cereal(s) added
6–7 months	Vegetables (puréed) added
8–9 months	Start finger foods (rusk, banana) and chopped (junior) foods
9 months	Meats, citrus juice (from a cup)
10 months	Egg yolk (cooked), bite-sized cooked foods
12 months	Whole egg, most table foods

Milk continues to be the main source of calories but a diminishing one. Sweetened fruit juices should be given by cup not bottle because the latter can promote dental caries. Infantile obesity is probably becoming less common in the United Kingdom now that people are aware of it. It is not usually caused by bottle feeding or early introduction of solids in themselves, but by more concentrated feeds, by pushing food at mealtimes, or by snacks in between. Between feeds, water for thirst and a minimum of snacks or sweets are good general rules.

Two other nutrients are not adequately supplied in all mixed diets. In communities where rickets occurs—for example, among Asian babies in northern cities—a supplement of vitamin D 10 μg (400 IU) a day is good insurance. In areas where the drinking water is not fluoridated, sodium fluoride prophylactic tablets or drops (0·25 mg/day) should be considered.

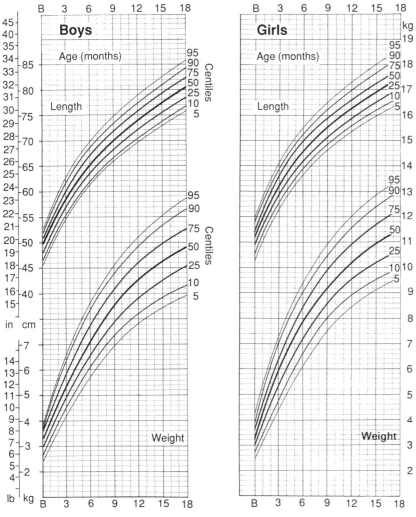

National Center for Health Statistics graph of percentile weights and heights for girls and boys from birth to 18 months, adopted by the World Health Organisation[11]

Ages by which babies had been given solid food (United Kingdom, 1985)[5]

Ages of babies	Percentages of babies given solid food
4 weeks	3
6 weeks	11
8 weeks	24
3 months	62
4 months	90
6 months	99
9 months	100

1 Department of Health and Social Security. *Present day practice in infant feeding: third report.* London: HMSO, 1988. (Report on Health and Social Subjects No 32.)
2 Department of Health and Social Security. *The composition of mature human milk.* London: HMSO, 1977. (Report on Health and Social Subjects No 12.)
3 Reeve LE, Chesney RW, deLuca HF. Vitamin D of human milk: identification of biologically active forms. *Am J Clin Nutr* 1982;**36**:122–6.
4 Howie PW, Forsyth JS, Ogston SA, Clark A, Florey C du V. Protective effect of breast feeding against infection. *BMJ* 1990;**300**:11–6.
5 Martin J, White A. *Infant feeding 1985.* London: HMSO/Office of Population Censuses and Surveys, 1988.
6 Palmer N. Breast-feeding—the Australian situation. *Journal of Food and Nutrition (Canberra)* 1985;**42**:13–8.
7 Anonymous. *Successful breastfeeding. A practical guide for mothers and midwives and other supporting breastfeeding mothers.* London: Royal College of Midwives, 1989.
8 Truswell AS, Dreosti IE, English RM, Palmer NP, Rutishauser IHE. *Recommended dietary intakes for use in Australia.* Canberra, Australia: National Health and Medical Research Council, 1991.
9 Yeung DL. *Infant nutrition. A study of feeding practices and growth from birth to 18 months.* Ottawa: Canadian Public Health Association, 1983.
10 Whitehead RG, Paul AA, Rowland MGM. Lactation in Cambridge and in the Gambia. In: Wharton BA, ed. *Topics in paediatrics 2.* Tunbridge Wells: Pitman (for the Royal College of Physicians), 1980:22–33.
11 Hamill PVV, Drizd TA, Johnson CL, Reed RB, Roche AF, Moore WM. Physical growth: National Center for Health Statistics percentiles. *Am J Clin Nutr* 1979;**32**:607–29.

6: CHILDREN AND ADOLESCENTS

Children

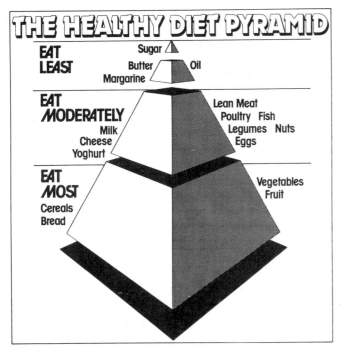

THE HEALTHY DIET PYRAMID

EAT LEAST — Sugar, Butter, Margarine, Oil

EAT MODERATELY — Milk Cheese Yoghurt / Lean Meat Poultry Fish Legumes Nuts Eggs

EAT MOST — Cereals Bread / Vegetables Fruit

Healthy diet pyramid (Australian Nutrition Foundation)

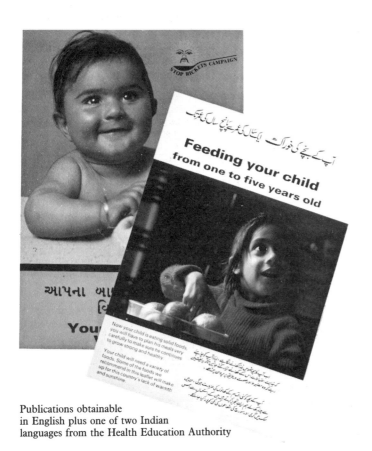

Publications obtainable
in English plus one of two Indian
languages from the Health Education Authority

What children eat is largely controlled by their mothers. Four simple principles should help them.

(1) Eat from each of the four basic food groups every day. These include all the essential nutrients between them.

(2) Aim for variety within each food group—for example, not always the same vegetable. The child should be prepared to eat food from other cultures. Faddiness is a social handicap in later life.

(3) To minimise dental caries, sweets and other sugary foods should be rationed and not eaten between meals as a rule. A healthy child going through a phase of not finishing ordinary amounts of food at three main daily meals should not have snacks between.

(4) Rickets is the most likely deficiency disease in Britain; children of people from the Indian subcontinent are most at risk in northern cities. The three preventive measures are:
- spending more time out of doors,
- eating plenty of the foods that contain some vitamin D,
- taking NHS vitamin drops (vitamins A, C, and D) in winter.

Foods that contain some **Vitamin D**

Milk, eggs, cheese, butter, liver all contain some.

Fatty fish (herring, mackerel, sardines, pilchards, tuna, and salmon) contain more.

Infant milks, infant cereals, margarines, some breakfast cereals, some yoghurts, and branded food drinks have vitamin D added during manufacture.

Faddy toddlers

After having a reliable appetite for their first 12 months, many children aged 1–3 go through a phase of poor eating, which can make parents anxious or even exasperated. Children are less enthusiastic about eating and refuse foods that the rest of the family eat, especially vegetables.

One reason for this is that growth slows at around 12 months. This can be seen in the changes in gradient of normal weight for age and height for age curves. It is even more obvious in weight and height velocity curves, which descend to about a quarter and a half, respectively, of the values in early infancy.

Advice for parents of faddy toddlers[1][2]

(1) Most toddlers will eat some form of bread, cereals, meat, milk, and some fruits and fruit juices. The fibre foregone in vegetables can be replaced by breads and the vitamins by fruits and juices.

(2) Don't have battles over foods. Don't use bribes or force. Try to avoid tension at meal times.

(3) Keep meal preparation for toddlers easy and quick, so you can accept it without anger if they won't eat what you've made for them.

(4) Make eating fun—for example, cut sandwiches, pieces of fruit, cheese, etc, into patterns. Let toddlers eat at a small table, etc.

(5) When it is clear that they won't eat any more, let them leave the table. Don't insist on clean plates; serve a little less next time. "With proper education, parents may be led to understand that a 'good' eater is not a big eater but a moderate eater".[1]

(6) If they want to eat a narrow range of foods let them; a monotonous diet can be quite healthy if it covers the main food groups and provides the essential nutrients.

(7) Don't give delicious (for them) high fat and sugar foods (cake or chocolates) before a meal *or* if they won't eat their main meals.

(8) Children are more likely to try new foods offered in small amounts at the start of meals when they are hungry. If they help preparing (or even growing) vegetable foods (for example, shelling peas or making salad) they may like to taste them.

(9) Many toddlers can't adjust to their parents' three meals but will eat nutritious foods as snacks.

Energy intake, which reaches an average of about 3·8 MJ/day (900 kcal/day) in boys at 12 months, is only about 4·2 MJ/day (1000 kcal/day) at 24 months.[3]

Other things are also happening. Children are discovering their independence and testing their choice in food selection. Once they have some control over what is offered, foods that they find unattractive are displaced by those they think delicious: cakes, biscuits, chocolate, crisps, ice cream, etc.

Schoolchildren

In the schoolgoing years 5/21 of children's meals during term time, or (including holidays) about 16% of their annual meals, are eaten at or near the school. The 1975 guidelines on school lunches of the Department of Education and Science aimed to provide about one third of children's energy needs and 42% of their protein needs. Other critical nutrients—iron, calcium, zinc, and several vitamins are associated with protein in the diet.

Since 1980, however, local authorities in the United Kingdom have no longer been obliged to provide school meals for most children, and the nutritional content of the food they do provide is no longer laid down.

In a nationwide survey of the total food intake (by 7 day record) of over 3000 British schoolchildren aged 10–11 and 14–15 the main foods consumed were (in descending order by weight): biscuits and cakes, meats (including beefburgers and meat pies), potato chips and crisps, breads, vegetables (including baked beans), fruits, breakfast cereals, confectionery, sugar, and fish. The main drinks were milk and soft drinks.[5]

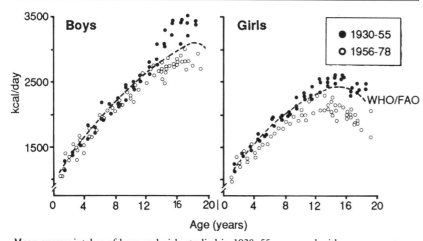

Mean energy intakes of boys and girls studied in 1930–55 compared with more recent studies in relation to WHO/FAO (1973) recommendations[4]

Adolescents

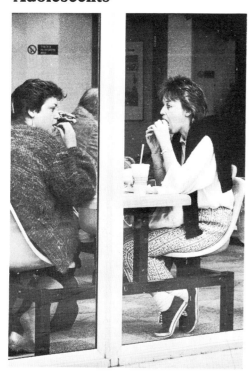

"Teenagers are not fed; they eat. For the first time in their lives they assume responsibility for their own food intakes. At the same time they are intensely involved in day-to-day life with their peers and preparation for their future lives as adults. Social pressures thrust choices at them: to drink or not to drink, to smoke or not to smoke, to develop their bodies to meet sometimes extreme ideals of slimness or athletic prowess. Few become interested in foods and nutrition except as part of a cult or fad such as vegetarianism or crash dieting."

E M N HAMILTON and E N WHITNEY[6]
Nutrition: Concepts and Controversies, 1979

Ten facets of eating behaviour are different or more pronounced in adolescents than in other people and each may cause concern in the older generation.

(1) *Missing meals*, especially breakfast. This does not usually affect classroom performance, partly because of—

(2) *Eating snacks* and confectionery. The major snack is usually in the afternoon, after school. Snacks tend to be high in "empty calories"—fat, alcohol, and sugar—but some provide calcium (for example, milk) or vitamin C (fruit).

(3) *"Fast," take away, or carry out foods*—These provide some nutritious portions, but adolescents may not choose balanced meals from what is offered. There is not enough accessible information about the nutrient composition of fast foods.

Children and adolescents

(4) *Unconventional meals* may be eaten in combinations and permutations that other members of the family do not approve of, but they often add up to an adequate nutritional mix.

(5) *Start of alcohol consumption*—This is the most dangerous of the new food habits. Alcohol-related accidents are the leading cause of death in the 15–24 year age group.

(6) *Soft drinks and other fun drinks*—If they are an alternative to alcoholic drinks soft drinks should not be discouraged, but they provide only empty calories and by replacing milk can reduce the intake of calcium.

(7) *Distincitive likes and dislikes for foods*—The order of preference differs between cultures and subcultures and between boys and girls.

(8) *High energy intakes*—Many adolescents go through a phase of eating much more than adults, sometimes up to 16·7 MJ (4000 kcal). This seems to occur near the age of peak height velocity in girls (around 12 years), but in boys may come later than the age of peak height velocity (usually 14 years). Presumably the larger, more muscular male late adolescent is expending more energy at this stage.

(9) *Low levels of some nutrients*—The critical ones are iron, calcium, and in some studies vitamins A and C and zinc. Iron deficiency is quite common in adolescent girls who are menstruating, still growing, and often restricting their food intake. It may sometimes occur in boys too. Accretion of calcium in the skeleton can be as much as 100 g/year at peak height velocity. Around 20% is absorbed so that about 500/365 g is neded in the diet—that is, 1370 mg/day.

Percentage of daily nutrients provided by different meals among 290 school students (boys and girls) aged 16–17 in Sydney, Australia (based on four day records and interviews)[7]

	Breakfast	Lunch	Dinner	Snacks
Energy	16·7	23·8	33·0	26·1
Protein	16	25	41	18
Fat	15	25	37	23
Carbohydrate	20	23	27	31
Alcohol	0	14	36	50
Calcium	26	19	26	28
Iron	23	23	37	9
Vitamin A	18	26	36	21
Thiamin	28	22	28	20
Riboflavin	27	17	26	18
Vitamin C	14	19	27	27

(10) *Adolescent dieters.* There are two aspects to this: obesity and social dieting. Obesity affects about 10% of boys and girls, but its exact prevalence is difficult to determine because there are no generally accepted standards for adolescents. Weight for age needs to take height into account and the stage of puberty. Obese adolesecents are usually inactive and tend to have low socioeconomic status. Dietary management should aim to hold the weight constant while the young person continues to grow and so thins out. Increased exercise should be emphasised and anorectic drugs should not be used.

Too thin: entering anorexia nervosa range*

Height without shoes		Weight (kg)
Metres	Ft, in	
1·45	4, 9	38
1·48	4, 10	39·5
1·50	4, 11	40·5
1·52	5, 0	41·5
1·54	5, 1	42·5
1·56	5, 1	44
1·58	5, 2	45
1·60	5, 3	46
1·62	5, 4	47
1·64	5, 5	48·5
1·66	5, 5	49·5
1·68	5, 6	50·5
1·70	5, 7	52
1·72	5, 8	53

*body mass index (W/H(m)^2) of 18

For every case of obesity there are several adolescent girls of normal weight modifying their diet because they are not as thin as they or their peers think they should be. Some may fast and binge alternately. With a smaller energy intake they are more likely not to reach their requirements for iron and other essential nutrients. In a small minority this social dieting goes on to anorexia nervosa (incidence in some places as high as 1% of middle class girls aged 15–25) or bulimia. Treatment of anorexia nervosa is best handled by a specialised team of psychiatrist and dietitian. The general practitioner's main role is to recognise the early case. The longer the duration the worse the prognosis. A young woman whose weight goes below a body mass index (weight (kg)/height(m)^2) of 18 should be warned, with her parents, that her thinness is unhealthy and referred for treatment if she cannot put on weight. By contrast, adolescent boys are more likely to worry that they are not growing tall enough or not developing enough muscles.

Does diet affect acne?

> "It is common practice today to believe that many teenagers have atrocious food habits and are on the brink of nutritional disaster. The basis of such a generalisation is questionable. We point with pride to our youth—their size, their attainments, and their vitality, even though we view with alarm their food habits. Are we implying that food has no relation to fitness, or do we have a distorted picture of their food choices and eating patterns?"
>
> R LEVERTON[8]

The popular belief is that chocolate, fatty foods, soft drinks, and beer can all aggravate acne vulgaris. This is not surprising since 85% of people have acne at some time during adolescence and most adolescents eat and enjoy these foods.

Controlled trials—for example, of cholcolate—have proved negative but their design can be criticised. It is very difficult to produce double blind conditions. Individual cases appear to respond to cutting down confecionery, fatty foods, or alcoholic drinks and there are other reasons to recommend such a dietary change. Zinc, polyunsaturated fats, and vitamin A are reported to improve acne, and adolescents can be advised to eat foods that are good sources of each: meat and wholemeal bread (zinc), polyunsaturated margarine or cooking oil, and carrots or liver (vitamin A).

Priorities

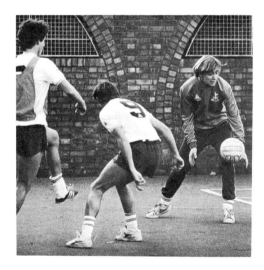

Perspective, patience, and a sense of humour help in watching and advising on adolescent food habits.

The serious ones are drinking with driving, usually in boys, and excessive slimming, usually in girls.

No young person wants to lose his teeth and spoil his good looks. As in children, sticky sugary foods should not be eaten between meals, or if they are the teeth should be thoroughly brushed afterwards.

Parents have more influence than they may think. They can choose which foods and drinks they buy and prepare and keep in the refrigerator. The adolescent's food habits were laid down in the family and the family remains one influence. The other three are the peer group, the need to develop an independent personality, and society in general.

Adolescence is a transitional stage when the structure of food habits is loosened. In a few years the young person will usually get married, work out a compromise set of food habits with the spouse or partner, and settle down to re-establish the eating behaviour of a new family. It is here, in preparing for and starting marriage that nutrition education should probably focus more.

1 Fomon SJ, Anderson TA, Stephen HYW, *et al. Nutritional disorders of children: prevention, screening and follow up.* Washington DC: US Government Printing Office, 1976:68.

2 Green C. *Toddler taming. A parents' guide to surviving the first four years.* Sydney: Doubleday, 1986.

3 Paul AA, Whitehead RG, Black AE. Energy intakes and growth from two months to three years in initialy breast-fed children. *Journal of Human Nutrition and Dietetics* 1990;3:79–82.

4 Whitehead RG, Paul AA, Cole TJ. Trends in food energy intakes throughout childhood from one to 18 years. *Human Nutrition: Applied Nutrition* 1982;36A:57–62.

5 Department of Health. *The diets of British schoolchildren.* London: HMSO, 1989 (Report on Health and Social Subjects No 36).

6 Hamilton EMN, Whitney EN. *Nutrition: concepts and controversies.* St Paul, Minnesota: West Publishing, 1979.

7 Truswell AS, Darnton-Hill I. Food habits of adolescents. *Nutrition Reviews* 1981;39:73–88.

8 Leverton RM. The paradox of teen-age nutrition. *J Am Diet Assoc* 1968;53: 13–6.

7: ADULTS YOUNG AND OLD

Young adults

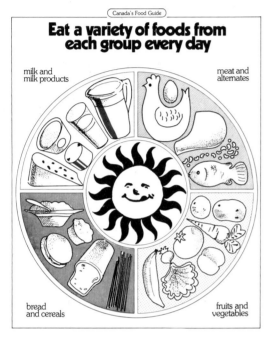

Food groups
Operation Lifestyle published by Health and Welfare, Canada

Adults should eat enough of the essential nutrients by eating a healthy varied diet. This is more difficult to achieve if people have a low energy intake and if much of their diet consists of fats, alcohol, and sugar, which provide empty calories but little or no protein or micronutrients.

The triple table shows three sets of recommendations, two by the DHSS and one by the United States National Research Council. These mostly give advice about how the part of the diet that provides energy—fats, carbohydrates, protein, etc—should be divided up. These dietary guidelines or goals give advice to the general public expressed in terms of averages. The average person, eating the average amount of (say) fat, should reduce this by or to a new national average. The advice has to be modified for individuals. Jack Sprat should not reduce fat intake as much as his wife.

There is much consistency and reiteration between the three sets of recommendations, though they were prepared by different committees from different viewpoints and given in different sequence. More regular exercise; less fat, alcohol, salt and sugar; and more cereals (preferably wholegrain), vegetables, and fruit are the recurring themes. The same themes appear too in contemporary dietary guidelines in Canada, Scandinavia, Germany, France, The Netherlands, Australia, and New Zealand.

Other aspects of a healthy diet, sometimes taken for granted, are that food should be wholesome and not contaminated with pathogenic microorganisms or their toxins or with other toxins (see chapter 15). Some of our foods are routinely enriched with micronutrients—for example, B vitamins in white flour, vitamins A and D in margarine.

The municipal drinking water should likewise be nearly chemically pure. Calcium, magnesium, sodium, and fluoride concentrations in it vary from place to place. There is suggestive—but not conclusive—evidence that hard water (more calcium or magnesium, or both), is associated with lower cardiovascular mortality. Fluoridation at 1 ppm is recommended by all orthodox medical and dental authorities.

Vegetarianism

Five grades of vegetarianism

(1) Don't eat meat of some animals (eg, horse) or some organs (eg, brain). *This is the norm for omnivorous humans except in a disaster*
(2) Don't eat meat but eat fish (and dairy produce). *Very little nutritional risk*
(3) Don't eat meat or fish but eat milk and eggs = lacto-ovo-vegetarian. *This is the most common degree of vegetarianism. The only nutritional risk is of iron deficiency*
(4) Don't eat any animal products = vegan. *Vitamin B-12 deficiency is likely and can be very serious in infants.[1] Adequate protein can be ensured with regular legume products and nuts. Calcium, iron, and zinc nutrition should be watched*
(5) Don't eat anything but fruit = fruitarian. *Unlike some primates, people cannot survive on such a diet for long and seldom try to. It is inadequate in protein and even sodium as well as the nutrients above*

Are vegetarians more healthy or less? The answer depends first on the degree of vegetarianism.

Vegans, who eat no animal products, are at risk of vitamin B-12 deficiency. Supplements are essential during pregnancy and for infants of vegans. Vegans lack the best dietary sources of calcium—milk, yoghurt, and cheese.

Lacto-ovo-vegetarians have no absolute nutritional risk. They miss the best absorbed form of iron in the diet, haem iron, but may largely compensate because ascorbic acid enhances the absorption of non-haem iron.

The other determinant is the reason for the vegetarianism. People belonging to long traditions of vegetarianism have the necessary recipes to prepare vegetarian centres for their dishes, using legumes (including soya) and nuts, and so have a good protein intake. It is new vegetarians, some of whom simply remove meat from the centre of the plate, who may eat inadequately.

On the whole vegetarians appear to have lower risk of obesity, coronary heart disease, hypertension, and cancer of the large bowel. However, many of the figures come from well documented groups such as Seventh Day Adventists, who have a more healthy lifestyle than average in other ways—for example, they do not smoke or drink alcohol.

Three sets of dietary guidelines for most adults

DHSS *Eating for Health*, 1979[2]	US National Research Council 1989[3]	DHSS *Diet and Cardiovascular Disease*, 1984[4]
Vitamin D supplements may be needed for pregnant, lactating, and housebound people. To ensure all the essential nutrients the diet should comprise a mixture of foods from five food groups: (1) cereals, (2) milk and dairy foods, (3) fruit and vegetables, (4) meat, fish, etc, [(5) fats and oils].† Avoid obesity by not eating more food than necessary for energy expenditure. Many people need to cut down on: *visible fats* (cream, butter, margarine, fat on meat, fried foods), *invisible fats* (in cakes, biscuits, puddings, pastry, ice cream), *and sugar* (in sweets, chocolate, puddings, soft drinks and beverages). Eat more bread, fresh fruit, and vegetables including potatoes. It would do no harm for most people to eat less protein. To eat less salt might be beneficial. Alcohol is not a necessary food.	Reduce total fat to 30% or less of calories and saturated fat to less than 10% of calories and dietary cholesterol to less than 300 mg/day. Polyunsaturated fatty acid optimal intake 7% to 8% of calories (not over 10%). Omega-3 polyunsaturates from regular fish consumption. (Concentrated fish oil supplements not recommended for general public.) Eat five or more servings of vegetables or fruits daily, especially green and yellow vegetables and citrus fruits, and six or more daily servings of bread, cereals, and legumes. Do not increase intake of added sugars. Maintain a moderate protein intake, not more than twice the RDA. Balance food intake and physical activity to maintain appropriate body weight. If you drink alcohol limit it to no more than two standard drinks a day. Women who are pregnant or attempting to conceive should avoid alcoholic beverages. Limit total salt intake to 6 g a day sodium chloride. Maintain adequate calcium intake. Avoid eating nutrient supplements with dose above the RDA (ie, avoid megavitamin suplements). Maintain an optimal intake of fluoride, particularly during the years of primary and secondary tooth formation and growth.	Eat less total fat: national averages should come down from 41% of calorie intake* to 35%. Eat less saturated fat: national average should come down to 15% of calories including *trans* fatty acids (which provide about 1·5% of calories). The polyunsaturated:saturated fat ratio may be increased to 0·45; polyunsaturated fat from 5% to 7% of calories. Intakes of simple sugars should not be increased (they are in fact falling). Alcohol intake over 80 g/day for men is harmful in general and may adversely affect the cardiovascular system; the effects of low or moderate intakes have not been adequately tested. Salt intake is needlessly high in Britain: consideration should be given to ways of reducing it. Compensate for reduced fat intake by increasing fibre-rich carbohydrate foods, eg, bread, cereals, fruit, and vegetables provided this can be achieved without increasing total salt or simple sugars. Obesity should be avoided or treated by appropriate food intake and regular exercise.

* Total calorie intake does not include alcohol in "Diet and Cardiovascular Disease" recommendations
† Many nutritionists think that the fats group for nutrition education should be pensioned off
RDA = recommended dietary allowance

The elderly

With aging (from 20–30 to over 70 years):

- Average body weight goes down after middle age (partly because of selective mortality of obese people).
- Lean body mass declines from average 60 to 50 kg in men and 40 to 35 kg in women.
- There is a loss of height and of the mass of skeleton.
- Muscle mass declines from about 450 g/kg to 300 g/kg.
- Body density goes down from 1·072 to 1·041 in men and from 1·040 to 1·016 in women.
- Body fat (as % of body weight) increases from about 20% to 30% in men and from 27% to 40% in women. It becomes more central and internal.
- Liver weight falls from about 25 g to 20 g/kg body weight.
- Basal metabolic rate goes down proportionally with lean body mass.

In Third World countries the children suffer most of the malnutrition. In Britain it is the elderly who are most at risk of nutritional deficiency, though this is usually mild or subclinical and often associated with other disease(s). But it is very misleading to lump everyone over 65 together and expect them all to show the same problems and diseases. Healthy elderly people who are socially integrated are no more likely to get into nutritional trouble than anyone else.

For most elderly people most of their life after 65 should be healthy and enjoyable. This "third age" is a time when people want to look after their health. They can now give more attention, time, and money to getting and keeping healthy. They can take plenty of gentle exercise, have none of the stress of the workplace, few deadlines, and plenty of rest, and have time to choose food carefully and prepare it nicely. The dietary guidelines for younger adults all apply after retirement.

(1) A nutritious diet from a variety of foods is more important than when younger because the total energy intake is usually smaller than in young adults. The number of calories needed is less but not the requirements for most essential nutrients.

(2) To be light in weight eases the load on osteoarthritic joints and aging heart and lungs and reduces the risk of accidents. Judicious regular exercise is much better than food restriction.

Adults young and old

Average daily intakes of elderly people in Britain (age 69-97)[5]

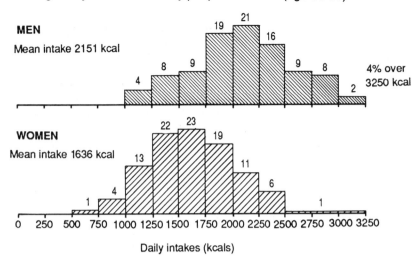

MEN
Mean intake 2151 kcal

4% over 3250 kcal

WOMEN
Mean intake 1636 kcal

Daily intakes (kcals)

> *DHSS* (1979)—In 365 elderly people living in their own houses 7% were diagnosed clinically malnourished and more showed subnormal biochemical tests.[5]
> *Vir and Love* (1979)—In 196 elderly people in Belfast institutions inadequate dietary intakes and subnormal values in biochemical tests were seen in substantial minorities.[6]
> *Morgan et al.* (1975)—Eleven biochemical tests of vitamin and protein status were performed in 93 acute geriatric admissions. In every patient at least one value was subnormal.[7]

(3) Cut down on fat. Fat supplies more empty calories than any other dietary component. It predisposes to thrombosis, raised plasma cholesterol, and atherogenesis.
(4) Eat plenty of bread and cereals (preferably wholegrain) and vegetables and fruit; older people are liable to constipation, and a good intake of fibre will help to control this.
(5) Limit alcohol consumption. The smaller liver cannot metabolise as much alcohol as in young adults and the consequences of falls or accidents are more serious. No more than one or two drinks a day.
(6) Cut down on salt and salty foods. They tend to raise blood pressure, and hypertension predisposes to strokes.
(7) Avoid too much sugar because of the empty calories, but dental caries is less troublesome in surviving mature teeth.

It is wrong, however, to use these guidelines for people who are declining in health (the "fourth age"); and some doubt even exists about whether low serum cholesterol concentration or body weight give any survival advantage to very old people.

Some suggested extra dietary guidelines for older people

(8) Women especially should keep up a good intake of calcium from (low fat) milk or cheese, or both. This may help to delay osteoporosis.
(9) Those who are housebound or do not get out regularly should arrange to take small prophylactic doses of vitamin D (5–10 µg/day).
(10) Old people should avoid big meals, as Hippocrates, Galen, and Avicenna all advised. On the other hand, they should not miss any of the three main daily meals.
(11) Coffee and tea in the evening may contribute to insomnia.
(12) There may be a place for fatty fish or small amounts of fish oils containing fatty acids like eicosapentaenoic acid (20:5, ω-3), which can reduce the risk of thrombosis. But this subject needs more research.

There have been several studies of the nutrition of old people in Britain and similar countries. Findings have differed, partly because different sectors of the elderly population have been sampled, partly because different parts of the range of possible biochemical tests have been done.

Nutritional deficiency is nearly always secondary to a social problem or to disease. The first step in diagnosing malnutrition is to recognise one or more *risk factors*.

The chances of risk factors and of nutritional deficiencies in elderly people increase progressively from those at normal risk (the healthy and socially integrated) through those with one or more chronic illness but who are nevertheless socially organised and the housebound to those at high risk—the institutionalised.

Social risk factors

Loneliness
Isolation
Immobility (no transport)
Poverty
Ignorance (the widower who cannot cook)
Bereavement
Alcoholism
Dependence
Regression

Medicial risk factors

Cancer and radiotherapy	Angina
Depression	Insomnia
Chronic bronchitis and emphysema	Blindness
Anorexia	Deafness
Cardiac failure	Paralysis
	Arthritis

Dementia
Gastrectomy
Sjörgen's syndrome
Diverticulitis
No teeth

Some common drugs that can lead to malnutrition

Aspirin and NSAIDs→ blood loss, so iron deficiency
Digoxin→ lowers appetite
Purgatives→ potassium loss
Cancer chemotherapy→ anorexia

Many diuretics→ potassium loss
Phenformin, Metformin →vitamin B12 malabsorption
Co-trimoxazole→ can antagonise folate

NSAIDs = non-steroidal anti-inflammatory drugs

Nutrients most likely to be deficient are (roughly in order of importance):

Total energy—thinness, wasting, undernutrition,

Potassium—deficiency can present with confusion, constipation, cardiac arrhythmias, muscle weakness, etc,

Folate—deficiency can present with anaemia or with confusion,

Vitamin D—deficiency can present with fractures or bone pains of osteomalacia

Water – frail old people may not drink enough, which can lead to urinary tract infection or dehydration

Dietary fibre—deficiency leads to constipation

Vitamin C—low plasma concentration, haemorrhages

Iron—anaemia, koilonychia

Protein—low plasma albumin, oedema

Calcium—low intake

Zinc—low plasma concentration

Thiamin—biochemical features of deficiency (red cell transketolase)

Magnesium—low plasma concentration

Vitamin A—low intake

Pyridoxine—biochemical features of deficiency

Assessment of nutritional status can be difficult in old people. The history of food intake may be unreliable because of poor memory. We are not yet sure whether the recommended intakes of some nutrients should be adjusted downward or upward, or by how much. Height may be impossible to measure exactly because of deformities. Weight-for-height standards (for younger adults) are not strictly applicable because of the decline in lean body mass.

Clinical examination is complicated by the presence of other diseases. Oedema is usually due to cardiovascular disease, loss of ankle jerks to aging nerves rather than nutritional deficiency. For several biochemical tests we are not quite sure what the normal range is in old people.

Preventive measures

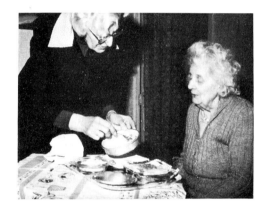

Only rarely are low intakes of nutrients and abnormal laboratory findings associated with a disturbance of function that would support the diagnosis of clinical malnutrition. The usual finding can best be called subclinical deficiency, and we are often not sure of its clinical importance. Exton-Smith considered it prudent to attempt to raise the level of nutrients to make people with subclinical deficiency more resistant to the effects of stress caused by non-nutritional diseases, which become increasingly common with advancing years.

General practitioners, with the younger family members or a friend, district nurse, or social worker can improve an old person's nutrition in several ways:

- suggest cooking lessons for retired men,

- arrange help for partly disabled women to adapt cooking techniques,

- organise delivery of heavy shopping,

- suggest (where there isn't one) buying a refrigerator or freezer,

- ensure that every old person or couple has an emergency food store,

- suggest that a younger relative helps with shopping and invites the old person for a regular good meal,

- arrange for him to her to attend a lunch club,

- arrange for meals on wheels,

- possibly prescribe micronutrient supplements, but some multivitamin tablets do not contain them all (they often miss folic acid) and there may be more need for potassium,

- build on established eating patterns when advising about changing food consumption; drastic changes are likely to confuse,

- warn that reduced sense of smell and sight make it hard to detect food that is no longer wholesome.

Diet for longevity

Claims that people live longer than usual in parts of Georgia, USSR or in Vilcabamba in Ecuador have proved dubious on investigation.

The food that our centenarians ate when young they say was less processed and simpler than contemporary food patterns. Of course it was. That was what ordinary people ate in 1890.

No special food emerged when a sample of centenarians recalled their lifestyles to the US House of Representatives Select Committee on Aging.

Nutrition in institutions

"Food, like sex, is one of the pleasures that stays with us all our lives" (as Alex Comfort puts it).[8] When life is limited because of disabilities and loss of social and environmental stimulation, it is very important for the morale and well being of old people in institutions that their food is what they like and served with courtesy and that they have at least some control over it. We younger adults are always making compromises between ideal nutrition and a little of what we fancy, and we must allow and help old people in nursing homes to do the same—by offering them a glass of sherry or beer, a favourite dessert, or a piece of confectionary.

In nursing homes, practices that contribute to poor nutrition include:
- lack of communication between nursing and kitchen staff,
- disregarding residents' suggestions about menus,
- ignoring residents' requirements for special diets,
- offering no choice of portion size or second helping,
- monotonous menus,
- not noting food left or residents not eating,
- not weighing residents regularly,
- little or no homestyle cooking,
- inadequate help with feeding frail residents,
- cooks lack basic knowledge of nutrition,
- meals rushed or served too early,
- no facilities for residents to make hot drinks for themselves,
- low fibre diets.

1 Wighton MC, Manson JI, Speed I, *et al*. Brain damage in infancy and dietary vitamin B12 deficiency. *Med J Aust* 1979;**2**:1–3.

2 Department of Health and Social Security. *Eating for health*. London: HMSO, 1979.

3 Committee on Diet and Health, Food and Nutrition Board, National Research Council. *Diet and health. Implications for reducing chronic disease risk*. Washington, DC: National Academy Press, 1989.

4 Department of Health and Social Security. *Diet and cardiovascular disease*. London: HMSO, 1984 (Report on Health and Social Subjects, No 28).

5 Department of Health and Social Security. *Nutrition and health in old age. The cross-sectional analysis of the findings of a survey made in 1972/3 of elderly people who had been studied in 1967/8*. London: HMSO, 1979. (Report on Health and Social Subjects No 16.)

6 Vir SC, Love AHG. Nutritional status of institutionalized and noninstitutionalized aged in Belfast, Northern Ireland. *Am J Clin Nutr* 1979;**32**:1934–47.

7 Morgan AG, Kelleher J, Walker BE, *et al*. A nutritional survey in the elderly: blood and urine vitamin levels. *Int J Vitamin Nutr Res* 1975;**45**:448–62.

8 Comfort A. *A good age*. London: Mitchell Beazley, 1977.

8: MALNUTRITION IN THE THIRD WORLD

1986–7 figures[1]	Average for 34 countries with lowest incomes (including China)	UK	People's Republic of China
Gross national product/head ($)	256	10 420	290
Population growth/year (%)	2·7	0·1	1·3
Infant mortality/1000	112	9	31
Under 5-year-olds mortality/1000	183	11	43
Calories available per head (% requirement)	92	128	111

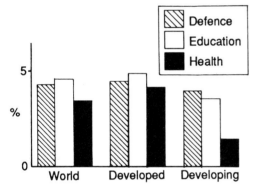

Expenditure on defence, education, and health as a percentage of Gross National Product, 1980[2]

Some former "developing countries" really have been developing. Countries like Hong Kong, Singapore, Korea, Venezuela, and Trinidad have joined the World Bank's upper middle income group, and as a byproduct malnutrition has largely disappeared. Other countries have been static or lost ground. In the table prosperity is compared as gross national product (GNP) per head. A country can become poorer from reduced income (caused by bad climate, economic mismanagement, or war) or from population growth faster than economic growth, or both.

About 3500 million of the world's total 5100 million people live in countries with low and lower middle incomes (on the current lists of the World Bank). In most of these countries people are very poor; the population is young and growing fast; there is no welfare state and little mechanisation. Food at an affordable price cannot be taken for granted; nor can clean drinking water. Tropical infections are an additional burden.

Public health indicators do not correlate closely with national income. The People's Republic of China is an outstanding example of a poor country which nevertheless has enough food to go round and a life expectancy better than that, for example, of Libya, whose GNP/head is 19 times higher. Economic development is thus only one factor—an important one—that reduces malnutrition. But even if a country's income stays low there are things that doctors, nurses, agriculturists, administrators, and politicians can do to combat malnutrition.

The diagnosis and management of malnutrition in Third World countries have to be mostly a public health operation. Many of the malnourished live in slums, shanty towns, or remote rural areas. They cannot be brought to a central teaching hospital. There are fewer doctors—in some countries only 1 for 50 000 people—so they have to work through teams of community health workers, who should be trained to recognise and cope with the common diseases, including malnutrition and the closely related infections.

Famine

Famines have been recorded frequently since 1708 BC (*Genesis*, xli) in many countries including England (last in 1812) and the severe famine in western Ireland in 1845. Notable famines associated with the second world war were in the Warsaw ghetto (1940), Bengal (1943), and West Holland (1944–5), and since then Bihar, India (1966), south east Nigeria (Biafran war 1968), Sahel (1972), and Ethiopia in recent years.

When there is not enough food for an entire community children stop growing and children and adults lose weight. The symptoms include thirst, craving for food, weakness, feeling cold, nocturia, amenorrhoea, and impotence.

The face at first looks younger but later becomes old and withered and expressionless; pupils react poorly to light. The skin is lax, pale, and dry and may show pigmented patches.

Hair becomes thinned or lost except in adolescents. The extremities are cold and cyanosed. There may be pressure sores. Subcutaneous fat disappears, skin turgor is lost, and muscles waste. The arm circumference is subnormal. Oedema may be present; in adults this is famine oedema, which is not associated with hypoalbuminaemia; it is different from the oedema of kwashiorkor. Temperature is subnormal. The pulse is slow, blood pressure low, and the heart small with muffled sounds. The abdomen is distended. Diarrhoea is common, often associated with blood. Muscles are weak and tendon jerks diminished. Psychologically, starving people lose initiative; they are apathetic, depressed, and introverted but become aggressive if food is nearby.

Malnutrition in the Third World

The two chief causes of famine are drought and war. There is usually a basis of chronic poverty. Disease of the staple crop is an occasional cause, as in the 1845 Irish famine (potato blight).

The present famine across Africa from Senegal to Ethiopia was precipitated by drought, but in this part of Africa population growth is very high and has outstripped food supply. The Sahara is advancing southwards because of overgrazing and there have been recurrent wars in and around Ethiopia.

Height (m)	Weight (kg)	
	80% of standard*	70% of standard
1·45	38	33
1·48	39·5	34·5
1·50	40·5	35
1·52	41·5	36
1·54	42·5	37
1·56	44	38·5
1·58	45	39
1·60	46	40
1·62	47	41
1·64	48·5	42
1·66	49·5	43
1·68	50·5	44
1·70	52	45·5
1·72	53	47
1·74	54·5	48
1·76	56	49
1·78	57	50
1·80	58	51
1·82	60	52
1·84	61	53·5
1·86	62	54
1·88	63·5	55·5
1·90	65	57

*Standard weight = W/H^2 22·5

In advanced starvation patients become completely inactive and may assume a flexed, fetal position. Infections are to be expected, especially gastrointestinal infections, pneumonia, typhus, and tuberculosis. The usual signs of infection (pyrexia, leucocytosis) may not appear. Delayed skin sensitivity with recall antigens—for example, tuberculin—are falsely negative. But the erythrocyte sedimentation rate is normal unless there is infection. Death comes quietly and often quite suddenly in the late stage of starvation. The very young and the very old are most vulnerable.

Inside the body plasma free fatty acids are increased; there is ketosis and may be a mild metabolic acidosis. Plasma glucose is low but albumin concentration is often normal. Insulin is diminished, reverse triiodothyronine replaces normal T3, and glucagon and cortisol concentrations tend to increase. The resting metabolic rate goes down considerably; oxygen consumption per person goes down more than when expressed per kg body weight. The urine has a fixed specific gravity, and creatinine excretion becomes as low as 300 mg/day. There may be a mild anaemia, leucopenia, and thrombocytopenia. The electrocardiogram shows sinus brachycardia and low voltages. All the organs are atrophied and have subnormal weights at necropsy except the brain, which tends to maintain its weight.

In the *management* of famine people need to be graded. In general:

Mild starvation = weight for height 90–80% standard (or W/H^2 20–18)
Moderate starvation = weight for height 80–71% standard (W/H^2 18–16)
Severe starvation = weight for height ≤ 70% standard (W/H^2 ≤ 15·7)

People with mild starvation are in no danger; those with moderate starvation need extra feeding. People who are severely underweight need hospital type care; 1500 to 2000 calories/day (6·3–8·4 kJ/day) will prevent the downward progress of undernutrition. Dehydration from diarrhoea may require oral or parenteral rehydration.

In severe starvation there is atrophy of the intestinal epithelium and of the exocrine pancreas and bile is dilute. When food becomes available the extra should be given in small amounts at first; food should be bland and preferably similar to the usual staple—for example, a cereal with some sugar, milk powder, and oil. Salt (NaCl) must be restricted, on the other hand refined foods may not contain enough potassium,[4] and a multivitamin preparation is desirable. A refeeding schedule of one month to put back each 5% loss of weight is a good guide.

Circumstances and resources are different in every famine. The problems are mainly non-medical: organising transport and repair of trucks and shelters, coordinating relief from different organisations, reconciling international workers with local politicians and administrators, arranging security of food stores, seeing that food is distributed on the basis of need, trying to procure the right food and the appropriate medical supplies. Civil disturbances do not occur during severe famine. They may happen at an early stage (food riots) or afterwards (revolution).

Meanwhile, the future has to be planned for; agricultural workers are going to be needed with enough strength to plough and plant the next crop when the rains return.

Protein-energy malnutrition[3]

Protein-energy malnutrition	Body weight as % of standard	Oedema	Deficit in weight for height
Marasmus	60	0	+ +
Marasmic kwashiorkor	60	+	+ +
Kwashiorkor	80–60*	+	+
Nutritional dwarf	60	0	minimal
Underweight child	80–60	0	+

*Occasional cases are not underweight at the oedematous stage

What is described here is malnutrition in children. Because children have higher protein requirements per calorie and are more at risk of being given a low protein diet, protein deficiency is more prominent in them.

In Third World countries around 2% of young children show severe protein-energy malnutrition and about 20% show mild to moderate forms. The World Health Organisation has estimated that about 100 000 000 children in the world at any time have moderate or severe protein-energy malnutrition. Though it affects only some children in each community it is a much larger and more intractable problem than famines.

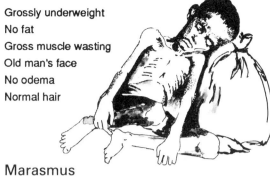

Grossly underweight

No fat

Gross muscle wasting

Old man's face

No odema

Normal hair

Marasmus

Oedema

Will not eat

Skin: patches of pigmentation and desquamation

Hair pale and thinned

Miserable and apathetic

Moon face

Liver usually palpable

Pitting oedema

Kwashiorkor

Nutritional marasmus is the commonest severe form of protein-energy malnutrition, the childhood version of starvation. It usually occurs at a younger age than kwashiorkor. The cause is a diet very low in both calories and protein—caused, for example, by early weaning then feeding dilute food because of poverty or ignorance. Poor hygiene leads to gastroenteritis and a vicious circle starts. Diarrhoea leads to poor appetite and more dilute foods. In turn further depletion leads to intestinal atrophy and more susceptibility to diarrhoea.

Kwashiorkor in its full blown form is less common than marasmus. It is most common in poor rural chidren, displaced from the breast by the next child and given a very low protein starchy porridge—for example, made with cassava or plantain. There have been several hypotheses about the antecedent diet because it is very difficult to reconstruct the exact dietary history of a malnourished child. But careful studies by Whitehead's group[5] of pre-kwashiorkor in Uganda compared with pre-marasmus in the Gambia, and other information support the classical hypotheses of protein deficiency with relatively adequate carbohydrate intake. Pure cases of kwashiorkor can develop in a few weeks and the patients sometimes have normal weight for age.

The pathogenesis of kwashiorkor appears to be: very low protein with more dietary carbohydrate leads to insulin secretion being maintained (unlike marasmus). Insulin spares muscle protein but causes loss of liver protein. So synthesis is reduced of two proteins made in the liver (*a*) plasma albumin, hence oedema, and (*b*) low density lipoproteins, hence lipids accumulate in the liver. Some of the features of kwashiorkor may be due to zinc deficiency.

Marasmic kwashiorkor has some features of both conditions. Severe protein-energy malnutrition can be thought of as a spectrum from marasmus to kwashiorkor. Most affected children have some skin lesions, hair changes, and fatty liver of kwashiorkor together with the wasting of marasmus. Malnourished children are likely to be depleted in other nutrients as well.

Treatment

Management of severe protein-energy malnutrition is in three phases.

(1) Resuscitation — Correction of dehydration, electrolyte disturbances, acidosis, hypoglycaemia, hypothermia, and treatment of infections.

(2) Start of cure — Refeeding, gradually working up the calories (from 100 to 150 kcal (420–630 kJ)) and protein (to about 1·5 g) per kg. There may be anorexia, and children often have to be hand fed, preferably in the lap of their mother or a nurse they know. Potassium, magnesium, and a multivitamin mixture are needed.

(3) Nutritional rehabilitation — After about three weeks if all goes well the child has lost oedema and its skin is healed. The child is no longer ill and has a good appetite but is still underweight for age. It takes many weeks of good feeding for catch up growth to be complete. During this stage the child should be looked after in a convalescent home or by its mother, who should if possible have been educated about nutrition and provided with extra food. Locally available foods should be used. Examples of nutritious combinations are given by Cameron and Hofvander.[6]

Other nutrients deficient in protein-energy malnutrition

Usually:	*In some areas:*
Potassium	Thiamin }—Thailand
Magnesium	Riboflavin }
Zinc	Niacin—southern Africa
Vitamin A	Iodine—areas of endemic
Iron	goitre
Folate	

Few reports also of:

Copper, chromium, vitamin K, essential fatty acids

Mild to moderate protein-energy malnutrition is much more common than the obvious severe forms. Outside observers, even the mothers themselves, do not notice most of these cases because the children are similar in size and vitality to children of the same age. The condition is like an iceberg. For every severe case there are likely to be seven to 10 in the community with lesser degrees of malnutrition. These latter children do not grow normally and are at increased risk of infection. They may also have more difficulty learning motor and cognitive skills.

Most children with mild protein-energy malnutrition are thin and underweight. Because scales are difficult to carry children who are malnourished can be most easily identified in the field by measuring the

Kwashiorkor

Marasmus severe and obvious protein-energy malnutrition

Pre-kwashiorkor eg low plasma albumin

Underweight children

The iceberg of malnutrition

Malnutrition in the Third World

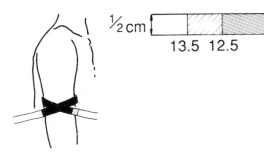

½ cm

13.5 12.5   0

mid-upper arm circumference. From 12 to 60 months of age over 13·5 cm is a normal circumference; 12·5 to 13·5 cm suggests mild malnutrition and under 12·5 cm indicates definite malnutrition. The normal circumference stays the same for the four years.

Measuring circumference of mid-upper arm

Sometimes a child is seen who has adapted to chronic inadequate feeding by reduced linear growth but he looks like a normal child a year or two younger—this is *nutritional dwarfism.*

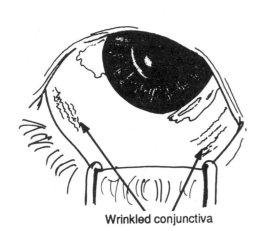

Road to Health card for Indonesia

Prevention of protein-energy malnutrition

Five measures to prevent protein-energy malnutrition are being actively promoted round the world.

Growth monitoring—The WHO has devised a simple growth chart—the Road to Health card. The mother keeps the card in a cellophane envelope and brings the child to a clinic regularly for weighing and advice.

Oral rehydration—The UNICEF formula is saving many lives from gastroenteritis: NaCl 3·5 g, $NaHCO_3$ 2·5 g, KCl 1·5 g, glucose 20 g (or sucrose 40 g) and clean water to 1 litre.

Breast feeding is a matter of life and death in a poor community with no facilities for hygiene. Additional food, prepared from locally available products,[6] is needed from 4 to 6 months of age.

Immunisation should be done against measles, tetanus, pertussis, diphtheria, polio, and tuberculosis.

Family planning advice and inexpensive or free contraception should be readily available.

Vitamin A deficiency and xerophthalmia

In 1857 David Livingstone first suggested that eye lesions in some African natives were caused by nutritional deficiency: "The eyes became affected as in the case of animals fed pure gluten or starch." The antixerophthalmia factor was the first of the vitamins to be isolated, in 1915 by McCollum in the USA. Xerophthalmia is a late manifestation of vitamin A deficiency. Its global incidence is estimated at some 500 000 new cases a year, half of which lead to blindness. Because of its social consequences vitamin A deficiency is given priority by the WHO for prevention programmes. The highest incidence is in east Asia—for example, Indonesia, India, Bangladesh, and the Philippines. It also occurs in some underdeveloped parts of Africa and Central and South America.

Wrinkled conjunctiva

Stages of xerophthalmia

Severe xerophthalmia is virtually confined to infants and young children and usually associated with protein-energy malnutrition. The stages are classified by the WHO as follows.

Night blindness is the earliest symptom but not elicited in infants.

In *conjunctival xerosis* one or more patches of dry non-wettable conjunctiva emerge "like sand banks at receding tide" when the child ceases to cry. It is caused by keratinising squamous metaphasia of the conjunctiva.

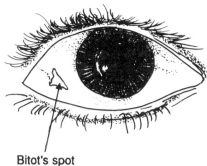

Bitot's spot

Bitot's spots are glistening white plaques formed of desquamated thickened epithelium, usually triangular and firmly adherent to the underlying conjunctiva.

Corneal xerosis is a haziness or a granular pebbly dryness of the cornea on routine light examination, beginning in the inferior cornea.

Corneal ulceration or keratomalacia—A punched out ulcer may occur or, in a severe case, colliquative necrosis of the cornea (keratomalacia). If promptly treated a small ulcer usually heals, leaving some vision. Large ulcers and keratomalacia usually result in an opaque cornea or perforation and phthisis bulbae.

Infants and children with xerophthalmia have a high mortality,[7] probably because other epithelia, respiratory and gastrointestinal, have lowered resistance to infections.

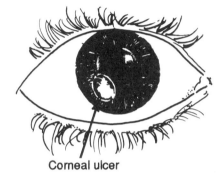

Corneal ulcer

Pathogenesis

In a classic experiment in Sheffield, British adult volunteers on a diet lacking vitamin A and carotene showed no deficiency effects until the second year of deprivation, and then they were minor (night blindness and follicular hyperkeratosis)—there was no xerophthalmia. British adult livers normally store enough vitamin A to last over a year. But in the Third World a different sequence can lead to severe deficiency:

● Low maternal intake of vitamin A and carotene and subnormal plasma retinol concentrations.

● Very low neonatal liver stores of vitamin (even in babies of well fed mothers liver vitamin A concentrations are about one fifth of the adult concentration).

● Low vitamin A and carotene concentrations in breast milk.

● Poor absorption and transport of vitamin A because of protein-energy malnutrition.

● Precipitation of clinical deficiency by infection(s).

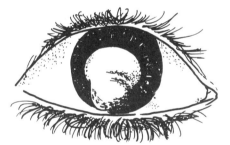

Perforation and prolapsed lens

Diagnosis and treatment

Xerophthalmia is extremely rare in Britain.[8] A British doctor going to work in a developing country should familiarise himself with the early features of xerophthalmia from colour photographs. (An excellent set is obtainable from American Foundation for Overseas Blind, 22 West 17th St, New York, NY 10011, USA. Or see *Control of Vitamin A Deficiency and Xerophthalmia*. Report of a Joint WHO/UNICEF/Hellen Keller International/IVACG Meeting. Geneva: WHO, 1982 (Technical Report Series 672).)

Treatment of xerophthalmia is urgent. The differential diagnosis includes smoke exposure, trauma, bacterial infections, measles, and trachoma. The child often has some other illness at the time like gastroenteritis, kwashiorkor, measles, or respiratory infection, which can distract attention from the eyes unless they are examined systematically. If in doubt a short course of vitamin A should be given. It can do no harm. Measles may precipitate or aggravate xerophthalmia in a malnourished child. In Cape Town a controlled trial in black children with measles showed a strikingly better outcome in those who were treated with vitamin A.[9]

The immediate treatment is 110 mg retinol palmitate or 66 mg retinol acetate (200 000 IU) orally or (if there is repeated vomiting or severe diarrhoea) 55 mg retinol palmitate (100 000 IU) *water soluble* preparation intramuscularly. For the next few days repeat the oral dose.

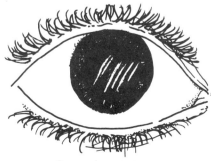

Scarred cornea

Malnutrition in the Third World

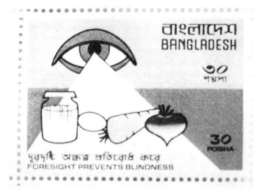

Bangladeshi postage stamp (palm oil, egg, carrot, etc)

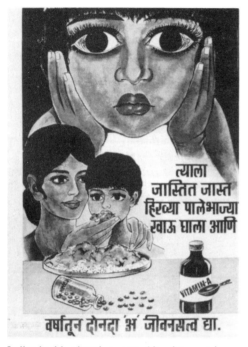

Indian health education poster (the plate contains green vegetables and orange-coloured fruits in addition to the staple, rice)[10]

Prevention

There are four strategies for prevention. In some countries two or more are being used side by side.

Nutrition education, emphasising garden cultivation and daily consumption of local dark green leafy vegetables, also of carrots, pumpkins, mangoes, red palm oil, yellow maize, and sweet potatoes, all good sources of pro-vitamin A carotenes.[10]

"Green vegetables are unbottled medicines" (E V McCOLLUM, 1925).

Vitamin A for mothers. The vitamin may be given to pregnant women, but it must not exceed 5000 IU (1 mg retinol) a day (ie the recommended nutrient intake) because more can be teratogenic.

Alternatively large single oral doses (200 000 IU) can be given to them in the first month after delivery. It should not be given later in case they become pregnant again.

Periodic dosing of young children in areas of high incidence with capsules of 110 mg retinol palmitate or 66 mg retinol acetate (200 000 IU) at six monthly intervals. A trial in Indonesia showed a 34% lower total mortality in young children given prophylactic vitamin A than in controls.[11]

Fortification of staple foods with vitamin A. In Britain margarines are fortified. In Central America sugar is fortified; in the Philippines fortification of monosodium glutamate (a widespread food flavour) is under trial. The World Food Programme requires dried skim milk used in its aid schemes to be fortified with vitamin A.

A regular newsletter, the *Xerophthalmia Club Bulletin*, edited by Dr D S McLaren, is sent free to anyone seriously concerned with xerophthalmia (address: International Centre for Eye Health, 27–29 Cayton Street, London EC1V 9EJ, England)

Iodine deficiency disorders (IDDs)[12]

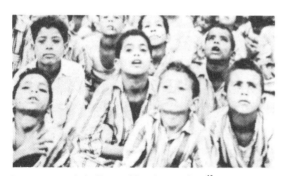

Boys at an oasis in Egypt. Most have goitres[13]

Iodine deficiency disorders are also given priority by WHO for preventive efforts among nutritional diseases because of their extent—they affect roughly 400 000 000 people—and feasibility of prevention. Their social importance is greater than it seemed.

In the major mountainous areas in the world—the Alps, Himalayas, Andes, Rockies, Cameroon mountains, and Highlands of New Guinea and on alluvial plains recently covered by glaciers—for example, round the Great Lakes of North America and in parts of New Zealand—the soil is lacking in iodine and so is the human diet if people rely on locally produced foods. When the iodine intake is below the minimum (about 50–75 µg/day) required to replace the turnover of thyroid hormones, pituitary thyrotrophin secretion increases and the thyroid takes up more than its usual 50% of absorbed iodine. Hypertrophy of the gland develops—that is, a goitre.

When just visible goitres occur in at least 5% of adolescents this is defined as endemic goitre. It usually shows first at puberty, and women are more affected than men. In some areas the iodine intake, indicated by the 24 hourly urinary iodine, is not very low and endemic goitre is attributed partly to thyroid antagonists such as glucosinolates or thiocyanate in certain brassicas or in cassava or soya beans.

When endemic goitre occurs in almost all the women a small percentage of babies, 1% up to 5%, are born with cretinism. There are two types. In nervous cretinism there is mental deficiency, deaf mutism, spasticity, and ataxia but features of hypothyroidism are hard to find. In myxoedematous cretinism there are dwarfism, signs of myxoedema, and no goitre. The nervous type predominates in Papua New Guinea and parts of the Andes, while the myxoedematous type is seen in Zaire.

Endemic goitre has by now almost disappeared from the low iodine regions of developed, industrial areas like Derbyshire, the North American middle west, Switzerland, New Zealand, and Tasmania because much or all the salt that people eat is iodised; foods come in to the area that were grown or reared on soils with normal iodine; iodophors used as disinfectants in dairies get into the milk; and iodate may be used as a bread additive.

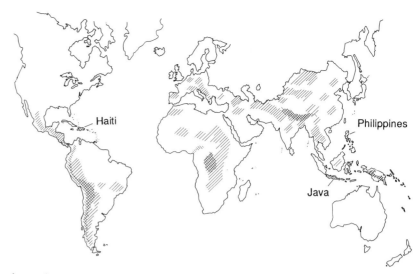

Areas of endemic goitre

But in many remote, inaccessible parts of the Third World endemic goitre and cretinism persist. Iodine status can be surveyed in such places by collecting single urine samples. Where goitre is common iodine excretions are all low and average less than 25 µg/1 g creatinine; the whole community is deficient. Endemic goitre was thought to be unaccompanied by functional effects (except for occasional local retrosternal pressure).

But in the 1980s it was recognised that "normal" people in goitrous districts (not diagnosed as cretins) have among them higher prevalences of deafness, slower reflexes, features of hypothyroidism, poorer learning ability, more stillbirths and malformed babies, and subnormal plasma thyroxines compared with control communities.[14] Any cretinism is thus the tip of the iceberg and the whole community on very low iodine intakes has a burden of miscellaneous impairments (iodine deficiency disorders, or IDDs) which reduce its capacity for productive work and development.

Iodised salt works only where there are roads and shops and a cash economy. For remote, isolated communities the first line of prevention is to inject all women of childbearing age with iodised poppyseed oil (lipiodol). One dose (1–2 ml) provides 475–950 mg iodine, reduces the goitre, prevents cretinism, and lasts three to five years. Boys up to 20 years are also treated. Iodised oil should not be given to women over 40 because in them there is a small risk of inducing thyrotoxicosis.

Iodine deficiency disorders (IDDs)

Endemic goitre—just visible goitre in at least 5% of adolescents

When nearly all mothers have endemic goitre 1%–5% of babies are born with one of two types of *cretinism*:

Nervous cretinism	—mental deficiency
	—deaf mutism
	—spasticity
	—ataxia
	—(features of hypothyroidism hard to find)
Myxoedematous cretinism—dwarfism
	—signs of myxoedema
	—(no goitre)

"Normal" people (not cretins) in goitrous districts, when compared with control communities, have:
- —higher incidence of deafness
- —slower reflexes
- —more pronounced features of hypothyroidism
- —poorer learning ability
- —more stillbirths and malformed babies

Other types of malnutrition

Anaemia—common world wide
Pellagra —seasonal in Third World maize (and some sorghum) eaters
—florid form rare
Beriberi —occasional in infants in parts of south east Asia

Nutritional anaemia is the other WHO priority. The commonest cause is iron deficiency, with folate deficiency second but well behind. Iron deficiency is probably the commonest of all nutritional deficiencies. It occurs in developed as well as Third World countries and will be considered in the next chapter.

Pellagra is still seen seen in parts of Africa where people subsist on maize, in black people in rural areas of southern Africa, and in Egypt.

Malnutrition in the Third World

It is also reported from Hyderabad, India, in people whose staple diet is sorghum. Sorghum eaters elsewhere in the world do not seem to be vulnerable. In Central America treating maize meal with lime ($Ca(OH)_2$), a traditional preliminary in preparing tortillas, makes the bound niacin available and prevents pellagra. In developed countries—for example, USA—maize meal is now fortified with niacin, and maize has been largely replaced by wheat in the diet. Pellagra is seasonal and the florid form is not common anywhere in the world.

Beriberi in adults has almost disappeared but infantile beriberi is still occasionally seen in some underdeveloped rural areas of South East Asia.

1 UNICEF. *The state of the world's children 1990*. Oxford and New York: Oxford University Press, 1990.
2 The World Bank, *World development report 1984*. New York and Oxford: Oxford University Press, 1984.
3 Suskind RM, Lewinter-Suskind L, eds. *The malnourished child*. New York: Raven Press, 1990.
4 Michaelson KF, Clausen T. Inadequate supplies of potassium and magnesium in relief food—implications and countermeasures. *Lancet* 1987;i:1421–3.
5 Whitehead RG, Coward WA, Lunn PG, *et al*. A comparison of the pathogenesis of protein-energy malnutrition in Uganda and The Gambia. *Trans R Soc Trop Med Hyg* 1977;**71**:189–95.
6 Cameron M, Hofvander Y. *Manual on feeding infants and young children*. Oxford, Delhi, and Nairobi: Oxford University Press, 1983.
7 Sommer A, Tarwotjo I, Hussaini G, Susanto D. Increased mortality in children with mild vitamin A deficiency. *Lancet* 1983;ii:585–8.
8 Olver J. Malnutrition in the Third World. *BMJ* 1985;**291**:897–8.
9 Hussey GD, Klein M. A randomized, controlled trial of vitamin A in children with severe measles. *N Engl J Med* 1990;**323**:160–4.
10 Oomen HAPC, Grubben GJH. *Tropical leaf vegetables in human nutrition*. Amsterdam: Koninklijk Instituut voor de Tropen, 1977.
11 Sommer A, Tarwotjo I, Djunaedi E, *et al*. Impact of vitamin A supplementation on childhood mortality: a randomized controlled community trial. *Lancet* 1986;i:1169–73.
12 Hetzel BS, Dunn JT, Stanbury JB, eds. *The prevention and control of iodine deficiency disorders*. Amsterdam and New York: Elsevier, 1987.
13 Davidson S, Passmore R, Brock JF, Truswell AS. *Human nutrition and dietietics*. 7th ed. Edinburgh: Churchill Livingstone, 1979.
14 Hetzel BS. Iodine deficiency disorders: a reappraisal of the problem of iodine deficiency with a view to its eradication. *Lancet* 1983;ii:1126–9.

9: OTHER NUTRITIONAL DEFICIENCIES IN AFFLUENT COMMUNITIES

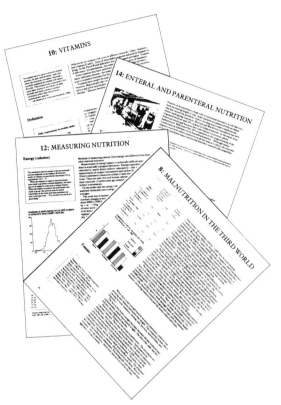

Protein-energy malnutrition in Britain and other Western industrial countries is almost always secondary to disease—for example, it may be due to diseases of the gastrointestinal tract (persistent vomiting, dysphagia, upper intestinal obstruction, malabsorption) or wasting diseases (some cancers, metabolic disorders) or to radiotherapy. It is briefly described in chapter 14 (Enteral and parenteral nutrition), where management to prevent or treat it in hospital is shown. How to assess the degree of malnutrition is dealt with in chapter 12 (Measuring nutrition). For a background, famine and childhood protein malnutrition are described in chapter 8 (Malnutrition in the Third World).

In Britain the vitamin deficiency that is still a public health problem is rickets. Its pathogenesis is discussed under vitamin D in chapter 10 (Vitamins). Among hospital patients in countries like Britain, however, the most common vitamin deficiency is probably folate deficiency, of which there is an account in chapter 10.

The most serious nutritional deficiency in alcoholics is the complex of Wernicke's encephalopathy and Korsakoff's psychosis, which is summarised under thiamin in chapter 10.

The following nutritional problems have not been discussed anywhere else in this book.

Iron deficiency

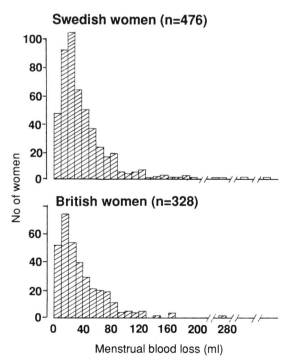

Menstrual blood loss in 476 Swedish and 328 British women[2]

Iron deficiency is probably the commonest nutritional deficiency in the world: according to one estimate it affects over 500 million people globally. In a survey in Vanuata, however, most people with hypochromic anaemia were found to have normal plasma ferritin but, by DNA analysis, a previously unsuspected high prevalence of α-thalassaemias.[1] Hypochromic anaemias in other tropical countries cannot all be assumed to be due to iron deficiency unless biochemical studies of iron status are done. People in industrial countries are affected as well as those in developing countries, especially women aged 15 to 50. Iron is the second most abundant metal in the earth's crust but it is virtually insoluble in the complexes of ferric iron usual in foods at neutral pH, and absorption is difficult.

There is no physiological mechanism for secretion of iron so maintenance of iron homoeostasis depends on its absorption. Normally in men, children, and postmenopausal women iron is lost only in desquamated surface cells from gut and skin at a rate of 1 mg/day or less.

Blood is by far the richest tissue in iron; 1 ml contains 0·5 mg so that a regular loss of only 2 ml/day—for example, from epistaxis or haemorrhoids—doubles the iron requirements. Women of reproductive age lose an average of 30 ml blood per period, corresponding to 0·5 mg iron per day, so they need more iron than men. An important minority lose considerably more, They, pregnant women, children growing fast, and anyone with chronic bleeding all need to absorb extra iron or use up what tissue stores they have.

Other nutritional deficiencies in affluent communities

Iron content of some foods[3] (mg/100)
(In descending order of total iron per usual serving)

Cockles (boiled)	26·0*
Black pudding (blood sausage)	20·0*
Liver, cooked: ox–pig	7·8–17·0*
Beef, rump steak, grilled, lean	3·5*
Lamb, leg, roast, lean	2·7*
Oatmeal	4·1
Legumes, cooked: peas–mung beans	1·4–2·6*
Green leafy vegetables: lettuce–spinach	0·9–4·0
Wines, red or white	0·6–1·2*
Egg, boiled	2·0
Dried fruit: rasins–peaches	1·6–6·8
Fish: cod–sardines (canned)	0·3–2·9*
Chicken, roast, meat	0·8*
Nuts: hazel–almonds	1·1–4·2
Chocolate, plain, dark	2·4
Potato, baked	0·8
Bread: white–wholemeal	1·7–2·5
Fresh fruit: pears–loganberries	0·1–1·4
Milk, cow's, whole	0·05

*Relatively high availability

Other foods with unusually high Fe content: Curry powder (75·0), Wheat bran and "All Bran" (12·0), some fortified breakfast cereals (20·0), duck (2·7), grouse (7·6), pigeon (19·0), hare (11·0), venison (8·0), heart (8·0), kidneys (8·0–12·0), sprats (4·5), cocoa powder (10·5), ground ginger (17·0), Bovril (14·0), black treacle (9·2), liquorice allsorts (8·1).

Absorption of iron is inefficient. It averages roughly 10% from a mixed diet but is much less from many plant foods and from eggs and dairy foods. Haem iron is better absorbed than non-haem iron. Absorption of the latter is enhanced by animal flesh and by ascorbic and other organic (eg citric and lactic) acids and reduced by tannins (as in tea) and phytates. Iron absorption is being studied by extrinsic labelling of foods with radioiron. The different factors in foods combine algebraically to produce a high, medium, or low absorption from the meal. For example, tea reduces iron absorption from a meal but orange juice enhances it.

Iron is essential for haemoglobin formation. It is also part of myoglobin, of some enzymes required for neurotransmitter synthesis, and of an important enzyme in DNA synthesis. In deficiency, sometimes even before there is anaemia, adults have decreased capacity for heavy work, pregnant women have an increased risk of low birth weight or premature babies, and children do not concentrate or learn as well as average.[4]

	Normal	Iron depletion	Iron deficient erythropoiesis	Iron deficiency anaemia
Iron stores				
Erythron iron				
Reticuloendothelial marrow iron (0–6)	2 - ≥3	0 - ≥1	0	0
Transferrin iron binding capacity (µg/dl)	330 ± 30	360	390	410
Plasma ferritin (µg/l)	100 ± 60	20	10	<10
Iron absorption	normal	↑	↑	↑
Plasma iron (µg/dl)	115 ± 50	115	<60	<40
Transferrin saturation (%)	35 ± 15	30	<15	<10
Sideroblasts (%)	40 - 60	40 - 60	<10	<10
Red blood cell protoporphyrin (µg/dl/RBC)	30	30	100	200
Erythrocytes	Normal	Normal	Normal	Microcytic and hypochromic

Sequential changes in the development of iron deficiency[2]

In people at risk of iron deficiency the haemoglobin (at least) should be checked, in:

- Infants at the age of 1 year
- Children and adolescents during phases of rapid growth
- Through and after pregnancy
- After gastric surgery at least once a year
- Women with heavy periods (direct questions may need to be asked)
- Patients presenting with gastrointestinal symptoms or disease
- Anyone with a history of recurrent bleeding, with a positive occult blood test, or a woman who is a frequent blood donor.

Ferrous sulphate tablets are standard therapy for iron deficiency anaemia, but it seems that patients often do not take all their tablets. Gastrointestinal side effects are related to the dose of elemental iron. Ferrous sulphate, three tablets a day (300 mg each), gives 180 mg of iron for the day. Compliance and hence response may be better with two ferrous sulphate or three ferrous gluconate (300 mg) tablets, which provide only 100 mg of iron per day. Slow release tablets are less effective.

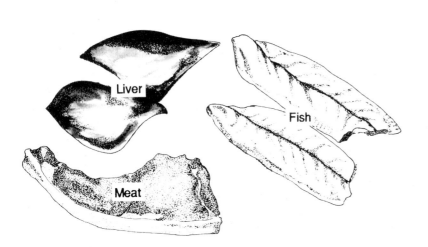

Prevention

A common cause of iron deficiency is that women, who require twice as much as men, consume only half as much. They often eat less liver, meat, and fish, the best sources of available iron. People who take no exercise or are on a weight reducing diet have such a low calorie intake that it is difficult for them to eat enough iron.[5] Iron absorption is increased in deficient individuals but this may not be enough to compensate for low intake or increased losses. Staple foods are fortified with iron in some countries (not in Britain) and old fashioned iron cooking pots add some iron to the food.

Calcium and the bones

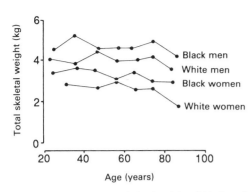

Age related changes in total skeletal weight of black and white people[6]

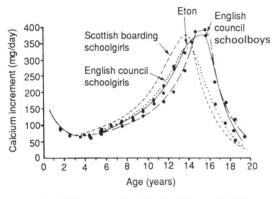

Estimated daily increment in skeletal calcium of children at various ages[7]

In 1927 a series of tests was carried out in Scotland in which about 1500 children in the ordinary elementary schools in the seven largest towns were given additional milk at school for a period of seven months. Periodic measurements of the children showed that the rate of growth in those getting the additional milk was about 20% greater than in those not getting additional milk. The increased rate of growth was accompanied by a noticeable improvement in health and vigour. This experiment was twice repeated by different observers who obtained substantially the same results on numbers up to 20 000 children.

ORR JB (LATER LORD BOYD ORR).
Food Health and Income, 1936.[8]

Other associations with osteoporosis

Obesity may protect but crash dieting increases urinary calcium loss.

Anorexia nervosa is associated.

Fluoridation of water supplies (1 ppm) appears to be protective.

High consumption of alcohol, coffee, meat, salt, and cola beverages tends to reduce available calcium.

Regular moderate weight bearing exercise may be protective.

Tobacco consumption and corticosteroid use increase the risk.

Calcium is the most obvious and persistent of the micronutrients, the fifth most abundant element (and the most abundant cation) in the body, yet it is more difficult to measure adequacy of intake for calcium than for other nutrients. There are two major questions about calcium. (1) Will a generous intake during childhood and adolescence contribute to taller adult height or heavier bones, or both? If so how much is needed?
(2) Will a generous intake from about 45 years onwards delay the onset of osteoporosis, especially in women, who are more likely to be affected? If so how much is best and in what form?

Over 99% of body calcium is in the skeleton. Here it not only provides structural support but is a large reservoir for maintaining the plasma calcium concentration at very stable concentrations. Any reduction of absorbed calcium does not show in the plasma concentration, which is immediately reset by an increased parathyroid hormone concentration and the formation of active 1,25 dihydroxyvitamin D (in the kidney from 25 hydroxyvitamin D). Ionised calcium in the plasma has many vital functions—muscle contractility, neuromuscular irritability, blood coagulation, etc—which would be disturbed if its concentration fell. By different modulators the ionised calcium inside cells is also tightly controlled. An inadequate dietary calcium will therefore not normally be allowed to lower plasma or intracellular calcium concentrations and their numerous important soft tissue functions; instead a little less will go into the bones in children or a little will be removed from the bones in adults.

Calcium in the bones amounts to 25 g at birth and builds up to about 1200 g in an adult. From the indices of growth and skeletal composition the amount of calcium which is being added to the bones each day in growing children can be calculated. It averages about 180 mg calcium per day but reaches 400 mg per day at the peak of adolescent linear growth. This amount is the required positive balance. Calcium absorption is inefficient—faecal calcium is often 70–80% of intake in adult calcium balances—and there is an obligatory loss of calcium in urine as well. The diet must therefore supply substantially more than the daily skeletal increment, and the recommended daily amount in Britain is 1000 mg in boys and 800 mg in girls 11–18 years. There is evidence that in some conditions a supplement of milk (the best source of calcium) has improved the growth rate of children. The great increase in the height of young Japanese adults from 1950 to 1970 coincided with a tripling of the national calcium intake from about the lowest in the world to 600 mg/day.

Yet it is hard to understand how poor children in the Third World on diets of cereals and vegetables and no milk obtain enough calcium to grow. Their final adult height is usually lower than in industrial countries, but osteoporosis in older people in less of a problem. There are four possibilities to explain the more economical handling of calcium in Third World people:
- More skin synthesis of vitamin D from sunshine in the tropics.
- Genetic selection.
- Lower intake of animal protein (which is known to increase the obligatory urinary calcium).
- Lower intake of salt (which also increases urinary calcium loss).

There have been some reports that metacarpal cortical width on x ray is greater after the menopause, or hip fractures less frequent in people who previously had relatively high calcium intakes,[9] although others have not found this. The effect may only be demonstrable in a population where some of the calcium intakes are low.

Urinary calcium loss increases at the menopause and an extra 200 mg over the premenopausal recommended dietary intake of 800 mg/day is estimated to be needed to maintain calcium balance.[10] Several clinical trials have shown a small effect of calcium supplementation on bone loss in menopausal women.[11] The effect is clearly less than that of oestrogens and appears to be more on cortical than trabecular bone. One trial suggests that the combination of a calcium supplement and low dose oestrogen might have a synergistic effect.[12] Longer term trials of calcium supplementation are needed, using modern high technology measurements of bone mass or fracture incidence as end points.

Other nutritional deficiencies in affluent communities

Moderate calcium supplementation with tablets is safe in the absence of conditions that cause hypercalcaemia or nephrolithiasis.

Dieting can be dangerous

Malnutrition can result from dietary regimens which happen to be very unbalanced nutritionally. Some of these were introduced by medical graduates, others are unscientific. The following are only a sample.

"Liquid protein" combined with fasting in the USA in the late 1970s led to at least 60 deaths from cardiac arrhythmias in people with no history of heart disease. The product "Prolinn," an extract from beef hides, lacked several essential amino acids. It was withdrawn, but prolonged fasting with or without protein supplements (even those of good biological value) carries the risk of sudden fatal arrhythmias and has been criticised authoritatively.

Zen macrobiotic diets consist of 10 levels. The highest level is 100% cereals and prescribes a very low fluid intake. These diets have led to scurvy and/or impaired renal function, anaemia, hypocalcaemia, and emaciation. In some cases these have been fatal. These diets have been condemned by the American Medical Association.

Dr Atkins's diet revolution—This weight reducing diet in a popular paperback written in 1972 prescribes a minimal carbohydrate intake. Ketosis is inevitable; and the diet raises plasma lipid concentrations. It was condemned by the American Medical Association but the book can still be found on bookstalls, having sold millions of copies.

Strict vegan diets for infants—Plant foods contain no vitamins B-12 or D. The latter can be synthesised in the skin if a child is exposed to sunlight, but the most serious nutritional complication of strict vegetarian diets is vitamin B-12 deficiency in infants. The milk of vegan mothers contains insufficient vitamin B-12 unless she takes a supplement. This vitamin is required for normal myelin formation, and infants' nervous systems are specially susceptible to deficiency. They can show impaired mental development, involuntary movements, and even coma responsive to vitamin B-12 as well as megaloblastic anaemia.

The Beverly Hills diet—This weight reducing diet requires consumption of nothing but fruit (all in a certain order and only the designated fruits) for the first 10 days. Some bread, salad, and meat are added later. The theory behind this diet is unscientific, and it has been criticised in detail in the *Journal of the American Medical Association*.

Articles which show the dangers of some diets

Liquid protein and fasting—Isner JM, et al. Circulation 1979;**60**:1401–12.

Zen macrobiotic diets—AMA Council on Foods and Nutrition. *JAMA* 1971;**218**:397–8.

Dr Atkins's diet revolution—AMA Council on Foods and Nutrition. *JAMA* 1973;**224**:1415–9.

Vitamin B-12 deficiency in vegan infants—Wighton MC, et al. Med J Aust 1979;ii:1–3 (see next box).

Beverly Hills diet—Mirkin GB, Shore RN. *JAMA* 1981;**246**:2235–7.

An exclusively breast fed infant of a vegan mother

"Neurological deterioration commenced between 3 and 6 months of age and progressed to a comatose premoribund state by the age of 9 months. Investigations revealed a mild nutritional vitamin B-12 deficiency in the mother and a very severe nutritional B-12 deficiency in the infant with severe megaloblastic anaemia. Treatment of the infant with vitamin B-12 resulted in a rapid clinical and haematological improvement but neurological recovery was incomplete . . ."

By 17 months of age his general level of motor, social, and intellectual development was that of a child of 11 months.

WIGHTON *et al*, 1979
(reference in previous box)

Eating disorders[13]

Anorexia nervosa is an illness of our time, although it was first described and named in 1874. Many teenage girls and young women say they are dieting to stay or become slim but most are not very successful. They do not stick to their diets. The young woman with anorexia nervosa is unusual: without talking about dieting she succeeds in losing a lot of the weight that the others say they would like to. But then she cannot stop. By rigid control of her eating she avoids foods that she understands to be fattening. She has a phobia of being fat and a distorted body image, seeing herself fatter than she really is. Amenorrhoea is characteristic.

Up to one in 100 middle class women from 15 to 25 may be affected. Before this loss of weight the young woman with anorexia nervosa was often a model of good behaviour, conformism, and achievement though this probably concealed a sense of ineffectiveness and self doubt.

Some women not only abstain: they have learnt to induce vomiting or purging and may have eating binges between. When habitual this behaviour is **bulimia nervosa**.

The physical effects of a young woman starving herself to 45 kg and below are similar to those described for famine in chapter 8. But there are differences. The anorectic patient (appetite is there but being suppressed) usually eats adequate protein and micronutrients and is restless and overactive. There is skinniness or emaciation, cold extremities, lanugo hair, bradycardia, low blood pressure, and normal pubic and axillary hair. Plasma potassium concentrations may be low if there has been vomiting or purging, and plasma cholesterol or carotene values are sometimes raised.

The amenorrhoea is similar to that which occurs in starvation.

Criteria for diagnosis

Anorexia nervosa
1 Refusal to maintain normal weight.
2 Loss of weight to body mass index* under 17.
3 Disturbance of body image.
4 Intense fear of becoming fat.
5 No known medical illness leading to weight loss.

Bulimia
1 Recurrent episodes of binge eating.
2 At least three of the following:
  (a) Consumption of high calorie, easily ingested foods during a binge,
  (b) Termination of binge by abdominal pain, sleep, or vomiting,
  (c) Inconspicuous eating during a binge,
  (d) Repeated attempts to lose weight,
  (e) Frequent weight fluctuations of more than 4·5 kg.
3 Awareness of abnormal eating pattern and fear of not being able to stop voluntarily.
4 Depressed mood after binge.
5 Not due to any physical disorder.

In practice intermediate forms are common

* Weight (kg)/height (m)^2

Other nutritional deficiencies in affluent communities

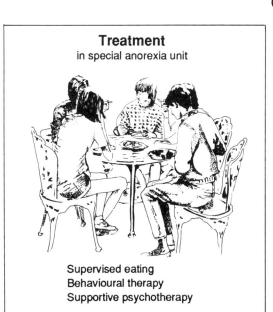
Early diagnosis is important because a long illness, severe weight loss, and bulimia (which tends to occur in older patients) are all bad prognostic features. The young woman denies she is too thin or that she is dieting. Amenorrhoea may appear to have preceded the weight loss. Other organic diseases that can lead to emaciation and amenorrhoea have to be excluded—for example, thyrotoxicosis, malabsorption, and hypopituitarism. But the bigger challenge for the family doctor is to detect the characteristic features of anorexia nervosa and to convince the young woman that she needs treatment.

Treatment is usually best managed by a specialised team, most often a psychiatrist with special experience in anorexia, working with a dietitian. A patient with anorexia nervosa of average severity should preferably be admitted to a special anorexia unit. The first aim is to persuade her to increase food intake and get her weight up to a target figure (usually a compromise). Eating is tactfully supervised by nurses, and behavioural principles can be effective: more privileges for each step of weight gain, previously agreed by the patient. As she is refed and becomes physically stronger it becomes easier for the patient to tackle the changes needed so that she can adapt to society and develop a healthier body image. Supportive psychotherapy starts in the unit and has to be continued as an outpatient.

Interactions of food, nutrition, and drugs

Nutrients, foods, and drugs can interact in several ways

- *Foods can affect drugs*, for example, by affecting absorption, an acute effect of single meals.
- *Nutrition can affect drugs.* Either the nutritional state or particular foods regularly eaten can affect drug metabolism and hence dosage and toxicity.
- *Particular drugs can affect the nutritional state.* Appetite, absorption, metabolism, and concentration of nutrients can be affected, positively or negatively, by different drugs (see below).
- *Drugs can cause unpleasant reactions to minor components in some foods* whose metabolism we normally take for granted—for example, hypertension from tyramine in cheese in patients taking monoamine oxidase inhibitors.
- *A few drugs are used as foods*, as part of the usual diet: alcoholic drinks, coffee, tea, and carbonated cola beverages.
- *Nutrients are used as drugs.* The nutrients are all obtainable in pure form. They may, in doses above the nutrient requirement, sometimes have a useful pharmacological action—for example, nicotinic acid for hyperlipidaemia.

Should I take the medicine before or after meals, doctor?

Most drugs are best taken *with or just after meals*, because this is the easiest way to remember to take any drug and some are gastric irritants. Absorption of several drugs is a little delayed but this is unimportant and a few are better absorbed when taken with meals—for example, griseofulvin, alprenolol, metoprolol, and labetalol.

Plenty of water should be taken with uricosurics (to prevent renal precipitation) and with cholestyramine and bulk formers like methyl cellulose.

A few drugs should be taken *half an hour before meals*: antibiotics which are labile in acid—ampicillin, benzylpenicillin, cloxacillin, erythromycin, lincomycin, tetracycline, rifampicin, and isoniazid. So should two antidiabetic agents—glibenclamide and glipizide—and, of course, appetite suppressant drugs.

Nutritional state can be affected by drugs

Particular drugs can affect the nutritional state, changing the results of biochemical tests or even leading on occasions to clinical undernutrition, overnutrition, or malnutrition.

Appetite may be decreased by anorectic drugs, bulking agents, dexamphetamine, phenformin, cardiac glycosides, glucagon, morphine, phenylbutazone, indomethacin, cyclophosphamide, fluorouracil, methylphenidate, salbutamol, levodopa, etc, and by drugs that alter taste (griseofulvin, penicillamine, and lincomycin).

Appetite may be increased by sulphonylureas, oral contraceptives, cyproheptidine, chlorpromazine, androgens, anabolic steroids, corticosteroids, insulin, lithium, amitriptyline, pizotifen, clomipramine, benzodiazepines, and metoclopramide.

Malabsorption for more than one nutrient may be induced by neomycin, kanamycin, paromomycin, colchicine, phenindione, para-aminosalicylic acid, chlortetracycline, cholestyramine, colestipol, cyclophosphamide, indomethacin, liquid paraffin (fat soluble vitamins), methotrexate, and methyldopa.

Energy metabolism may be stimulated by caffeine, smoking, and some sympathomimetic drugs.

Carbohydrates—Increased blood glucose concentrations may be produced by corticosteroids, thiazide diuretics, diazoxide, oral contraceptives, and phenytoin. Hypoglycaemia may be produced by propranolol and by alcohol (as well as by sulphonylureas, biguanides, and insulin).

Lipids—*Plasma total cholesterol* may be raised by chlorpromazine and some oral contraceptives. As well as specific cholesterol lowering drugs, aspirin, para-aminosalicylic acid, colchicine, trifluperidol, phenformin, and sulphinpyrazone may lower total cholesterol. *Plasma high density lipoprotein cholesterol* may be raised by phenytoin, ethanol, cimetidine, terbutaline, and prazosin. It may be lowered by danazol, propranolol, and oxprenolol.

Plasma triglycerides may be raised by propranolol, ethanol, and (oestrogenic) oral contraceptives. They may be lowered by norethisterone.

Protein–Nitrogen balance may be made negative by corticosteroids, vaccines, and tetracyclines. It may be made positive by insulin or anabolic steroids. *Plasma amino acids* may be increased by tranylcypromine and lowered by oral contraceptives. Plasma phenylalanine may be raised by trimethoprim and methotrexate.

Thiamin absorption can be reduced by ethanol or by antacids,

Riboflavin status may be lowered by oral contraceptives and by chlorpromazine.

Niacin may be antagonised by isoniazid.

Vitamin B-6 may be antagonised by isoniazid, hydralazine, cycloserine, ethionamide, penicillamine, oral contraceptives, oestrogens, hydrocortisone, imipramine, levodopa, piperazine, and pyrazinamide.

Folate may be antagonised by ethanol, phenytoin, oral contaceptives (uncommonly), cycloserine, triamterene, and cholestyramine. In addition

Other nutritional deficiencies in affluent communities

several drugs owe their antibacterial action to antagonism of folate metabolism—more in microbial than mammalian cells—pyrimethamine, trimethoprim, and pentamidine. Methotrexate, aminopterin, and methotrexate are potent folate antagonists which have more effect on rapidly dividing cells—for example, cancer cells.

Vitamin B-12 absorption may be impaired by slow K, para-aminosalicylic acid, metformin, colchicine, trifluoperazine, and by high doses of vitamin C, cholestyramine, and methotrexate. Prolonged nitrous oxide anaesthesia oxidises vitamin B-12 in vivo. Smoking and oral contraceptives reduce the plasma concentration.

Vitamin C—Plasma concentrations are lowered by oral contraceptives, smoking, aspirin, and tetracycline. Ascorbate excretion is increased by corticosteroids, phenylbutazone, sulphinpyrazone, and chlorcyclizine.

Vitamin A plasma concentration is increased by oral contraceptives. Absorption may be reduced by liquid paraffin and cholestyramine.

Vitamin D status is lowered by anticonvulsants—for example, phenytoin, phenobarbitone, glutethimide, and when these are taken in high dose for long periods rickets can occur.

Vitamin E is antagonised by iron in premature newborns.

Vitamin K—Coumarin drugs—for example, warfarin—are antimetabolites. Purgatives and intestinal antibiotics, such as neomycin, tetracyclines, and sulphonamides, may remove the contribution from colonic bacteria. Salicylates and cholestyramine may reduce absorption, and cefoperazone antagonises the vitamin K-epoxide cycle.

Potassium—Drugs are important causes of potassium depletion: purgatives and laxatives increase faecal loss; thiazide diuretics and frusemide and ethacrynic acid increase renal loss. Other drugs that may increase urinary potassium are carbenicillin, penicillin, glucocorticoids, liquorice, outdated tetracycline, gentamicin, and alcohol.

Calcium—Absorption may be increased by aluminium hydroxide or by cholestyramine and decreased by phosphates and corticosteroids. Thiazide diuretics decrease urinary calcium excretion. Gentamicin, mithramycin, actinomycin D, and ethacrynic acid increase it.

Iron—Allopurinol, fructose, and ascorbic acid increase absorption. Antacids, phosphates, and tetracycline decrease it. Oral contraceptives tend to increase serum iron.

Iodine—Sulphonylureas, phenylbutazone, para-aminosalicylic acid, cobalt, and lithium can cause goitre; they interfere with iodine uptake in the gland. Serum protein bound iodine is increased by oral contraceptives, *x* ray contrast media, and potassium iodide, and decreased by phenytoin.

Phosphate absorption is decreased by aluminium and calcium compounds.

Zinc depletion from increased urinary excretion may be produced by thiazide diuretics and frusemide, by cisplatin, penicillamine, and alcohol.

Magnesium depletion from increased urinary loss may be produced by thiazides and frusemide, cisplatin, alcohol, aminoglycosides, amphotericin, cyclosporin, and gentamicin.

1 Bowden DK, Hill AVS, Higgs DR, Weatherall DJ, Clegg JB. Relative roles of genetic factors, dietary deficiency, and infection in anaemia in Vanuatu, south-west Pacific. *Lancet* 1985;ii:1025–8.
2 Bothwell TH, Charlton RW, Cook JD, Finch CA. *Iron metabolism in man.* Oxford: Blackwell, 1979:251.
3 Paul AA, Southgate DAT. *McCance and Widdowson's the composition of foods.* 4th ed. London: HMSO, 1978.
4 Dallman PR. Iron deficiency: does it matter? *J Intern Med* 1989;**226**:367–72.
5 Barber SA, Bull NL, Buss DH. Low iron intakes among young women in Britain. *BMJ* 1985;**290**:7443–4.
6 Merz AL, Trotter M, Peterson RR. Estimation of skeletal weight in the living. *Am J Phys Anthropol* 1956;**14**:589–610.
7 Leitch I, Aitken FC The estimation of calcium requirements: a re-examination. *Nutr Rev* 1959;**29**:393–407.

8 Orr JB. *Food, health and income. Report on a survey of adequacy of diet in relation to income.* London: Macmillan, 1936.
9 Holbrook TL, Barret-Connor E, Wingard DL. Dietary calcium and risk of hip fractures: 14 year prospective population study. *Lancet* 1988;ii:1046–9.
10 Truswell AS, Dreosti IE, English RM, Palmer NP, Rutishauser IHE. *Recommended nutrient intakes: Australian papers.* Mosman, New South Wales: Australian Professional Publications, 1990.
11 Nordin BEC, Heaney RP. Calcium supplementation of the diet: justified by present evidence. *BMJ* 1990;**300**:1056–60.
12 Ettinger B, Genant HK, Cann CE. Postmenopausal bone loss is prevented by treatment with low-dosage estrogen with calcium. *Ann Intern Med* 1987;**106**:40–5.
13 Beumont PJV, Burrows GD, Casper RC, eds. *Handbook of eating disorders. Part I. Anorexia and bulimia nervosa.* Amsterdam: Elsevier, 1987.

10: VITAMINS

"No animal can live upon a mixture of pure protein, fat and carbohydrate, and even when the necessary inorganic material is carefully supplied the animal still cannot flourish. The animal body is adjusted to live upon plant tissues or the tissues of other animals and these contain countless substances other than the proteins, carbohydrates and fats."
SIR FREDERICK GOWLAND HOPKINS (1906)

Deficiencies of vitamins still occur in affluent countries: folate, thiamin and vitamins D and C. Some of these deficiencies are induced by diseases or drugs. In the Third World deficiency diseases are more prevalent. Vitamin A deficiency (xerophthalmia), for example, is a major cause of blindness.

Some vitamins may have useful actions above the dose that prevents classic deficiency disease—for example, vitamins A, C, and B-6; nicotinic acid is a standard treatment for hyperlipidaemia.

Vitamins have caught the popular imagination, and they are also big business. Many people take over the counter vitamins without medical advice and a few unorthodox practitoners prescribe "megavitamin therapy." Doctors therefore need to know the symptoms of overdosage.

Definition

Vitamins are:
(a) Organic substances or groups of related substances;
(b) found in some foods;
(c) substances with specific biochemical functions in the human body
(d) not made in the body (or not in sufficient quantity), and
(e) required in *very small* amounts.

Many people seem to have lost sight of point (e), but it appears in all dictionary definitions and can be seen in the table of requirements. The daily requirement of most vitamins is around 1 mg, the weight of one grain of raw sugar. There are no exceptions to points (a), (b), and (e). On point (c), the biochemical action of most vitamins can now be visualised, but those of vitamins A and C are not yet explained fully, and the active metabolite of vitamin D acts as a hormone. Exceptions to point (d) are that certain carotenoids can replace vitamin A; proteins (through the amino acid, tryptophan) can replace niacin; and exposure to sunlight can replace vitamin D.

Daily requirements for healthy adults

Vitamin A	1 mg
Thiamin	1 mg
Riboflavin	1·5 mg
Niacin	15–20 mg*
Vitamin B-6	3 mg
Pantothenic acid	5 mg
Biotin	100 µg
Folate	200 µg†
Vitamin B-12	3 µg
Vitamin C	30–60 mg
Vitamin D	3 µg‡
Vitamin E	10 mg
Vitamin K	100 µg

* Part replaceable by tryptophan in proteins.
† Double this in pregnancy.
‡ More for growth; no dietary requirement if adequate exposure to sunlight.

Recommended names for vitamins

Recommended name*	Alternative name	Usual pharmaceutical preparation
Vitamin A	Retinol	Retinol palmitate
Thiamin	Vitamin B$_1$	Thiamin hydrochloride
Riboflavin	Vitamin B$_2$	Riboflavin
Niacin	Nicotinic acid and nicotinamide	Nicotinamide
Vitamin B-6	Pyridoxine	Pyridoxine hydrochloride
Pantothenic acid		Calcium pantothenate
Biotin		Biotin
Folate	Folacin	Folic acid
Vitamin B-12	Cobalamin	Cyanocobalamin or hydroxocobalamin
Vitamin C	Ascorbic acid	Ascorbic acid
Vitamin D	Vitamins D$_2$ and D$_3$	(Ergo) calciferol
Vitamin E		α-Tocopherol
Vitamin K		Vitamin K$_1$

* International Union of Nutritional Sciences

Vitamins

Vitamin A

Food sources of vitamin A

Preformed vitamin A

Liver, fish liver oils,

kidney, dairy produce,

eggs, eel, fortified margarine

β Carotene

Carrots, red palm oil,

dark green leafy vegetables

(spinach, broccoli, sprouts, etc),

apricots, melon, pumpkin

In Britain on average 34% comes from liver, 24% from vegetables, and 14% from milk and its products

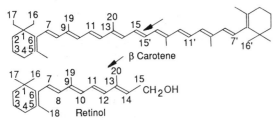

Formation of retinol from β carotene

Best understood of the actions of vitamin A is its role in night vision; 11-*cis* retinaldehyde is combined with a specific protein in the light-sensitive pigment, rhodopsin, in the rods of the retina. Night blindness occurs in children deficient in vitamin A in some Third World countries, and in affuent countries it is seen rarely in patients with chronic biliary obstruction or malabsorption.

Vitamin A also has important effects in mucus secreting epithelia. The classical effect of deficiency is xerophthalmia. Glycoprotein synthesis is impaired and there is metaplasia of the conjunctiva and cornea. The corneal damage is estimated to cause 500 000 new cases of blindness a year in children in South East Asia. Prevention is by giving foods that contain β carotene—for example, mangoes, pumpkins, or dark green vegetables—or six monthly high dose (60 mg) capsules of vitamin A. Other epithelia, such as in the respiratory tract, and the bones are also affected in less florid ways, and mortality, usually attributed to infections, is high in children with xerophthalmia.

Preformed vitamin A (retinol) is found in animal foods: liver is the richest source, but about two thirds of vitamin A intake in Britain comes from carotenes, yellow and orange pigments in the leaves of vegetables and in some fruits, chiefly β carotene. One molecule of β carotene can be cleaved by a specific intestinal enzyme into two molecules of vitamin A. But this conversion is not very efficient, 6 μg β carotene is assumed to be equivalent to 1 μg retinol. Vitamin A is stored in the liver; stores are enough for one to two years in most British adults. Retinol is transported from the liver to the rest of the body on retinol binding protein, part of the pre-albumin complex. Its concentration does not reflect vitamin A intake except when this is very low or high.

Epidemiological evidence suggests that vitamin A or carotene, or both, may protect against some epithelial cancers, such as bronchial cancers, but the data are not fully consistent. Large doses of retinoids have slowed progression of some skin cancers but this may be a different type of action. The US National Research Council's committee on diet, nutrition, and cancer recommends that people should increase their consumption of vegetables and fruit.

In supranutritional amounts vitamin A reduces both keratinisation of skin and sebum production. New retinoids, retinol derivatives synthesised by organic chemists, are more effective and less toxic. 13-*cis* retinoic acid and its aromatic analogue, etretinate, are effective in severe acne and in psoriasis. They should not be used, however, in women who are likely to become pregnant because they are teratogenic.

Over 500 cases of vitamin A intoxication have been reported in nearly 200 separate reports. A man's death in Croydon in 1974 from liver cirrhosis was presumably due to massive self medication with vitamin A. Acute effects of hypervitaminosis A are raised intracranial pressure and skin desquamation. Chronic overdose, which can occur with only 10 times the recommended nutrient intake, causes liver damage, skin changes, and exostoses. A high plasma vitamin A concentration confirms the diagnosis. High intakes of carotene, on the other hand, colour the plasma and skin (hypercarotenaemia) but do not appear to be dangerous.

Thiamin (vitamin B₁)

Food sources of thiamin

Whole wheat

wheat germ (richest source)

yeast, pulses, nuts

pork, duck, Marmite

oatmeal

fortified breakfast cereals

cod's roe

other meats

In Britain on average 42% comes from all cereals combined

Thiamin plays a part in the metabolism of carbohydrates, alcohol, and branched chain amino acids. The body contains only 30 mg—30 times the daily nutrient requirement—and deficiency starts after about a month, sooner on a thiamin free diet than for any other vitamin. The requirements are proportional to the non-fat energy intake. The two principal deficiency diseases are beriberi and Wernicke-Korsakoff syndrome.

Beriberi is now rare in the countries where it was originally described—Japan, Indonesia, and Malaysia. In Western countries occasional cases are seen in alcoholics: clinical features are a high output cardiac failure with few electrocardiographic changes and a prompt response to thiamin treatment alone.

Wernicke-Korsakoff syndrome

In 1880 Wernicke first described an encephalopathy.
Characteristic features are:
- Ophthalmoplegia (lateral or vertical)
- Nystagmus
- Stupor or apathy
- Ataxia

With treatment most patients pass through a phase in which they show the memory disorder, first described by Korsakoff (1887), which consists of inability to retain new memories and confabulation.

The pathological findings in Wernicke's encephalopathy and Korsakoff's psychosis are similar: capillary haemorrhages in the mamillary bodies and round the aqueduct in the mid brain.

Wernicke's encephalopathy responds rapidly to thiamin but Korsakoff's psychosis responds slowly or not at all.

Wernicke-Korsakoff syndrome is usually seen in alcoholics: it occurs occasionally in people who fast (such as hunger strikers) or who have persistent vomiting (as in hyperemesis gravidarum). Early recognition is important. The ophthalmoplegia and lowered consciousness respond to thiamin (50 mg intramuscularly) in two days, but if treatment is delayed the memory may never recover. Red cell transketolase and the effect on it of thiamin pyrophosphate in vitro are used to confirm thiamin deficiency, but fresh whole blood is needed and the test must be performed before thiamin treatment is started. If thiamin deficiency is suspected treatment should be started without waiting for the laboratory result. Two days later there will either have been a clinical response and a positive laboratory report or the provisional diagnosis will not have been confirmed.

Patients on regular haemodialysis should routinely be given small supplements of thiamin and other water soluble vitamins. Thiamin should also be given prophylactically to people with persistent vomiting or prolonged gastric aspiration and those who go on long fasts. The toxicity of thiamin is very low, though occasional cases of anaphylaxis have been reported after intravenous injection.

Riboflavin (vitamin B$_2$)

Food sources of riboflavin

Liver, kidney (richest source)

Milk, yoghurt,

cheese, Marmite,

eggs, wheat germ,

wheat bran,

mushrooms,

fortified cereals

In Britain on average milk and cheese supply 41%

Riboflavin has a vital role in cellular oxidation. Its biochemical functions do not easily explain the clinical manifestations that have been recorded in volunteers on a riboflavin deficient diet: angular stomatitis, cheilosis, atrophic papillae on the tongue, nasolabial dyssebacea, and anaemia. There are no real body stores of riboflavin, but the liver contains enough (in coenzyme form) to withstand depletion for about three months.

Most of the features of riboflavin deficiency have more than one cause. Angular stomatitis, for example, may occur with deficiencies of niacin, pyridoxine, or iron; after herpes febrilis; or with ill fitting dentures. Clinical riboflavin deficiency is very uncommon in milk drinking countries like Britain. Pregnant women, people with thyrotoxicosis, and those taking chlorpromazine, imipramine, and amitriptyline have increased requirements. Riboflavin has to be included in infant formulas, fluids for total parenteral nutrition, and supplements for patients on dialysis.

Niacin

Food sources of niacin

Liver, kidney (richest source)

meat, poultry

fish

brewer's yeast, Marmite,

peanuts

bran, pulses

wholemeal wheat

coffee

In Britain on average all meats and products supply 35%

Niacin (nicotinamide and nicotinic acid) is the part of the coenzymes, nicotinamide adenine dinucleotide (NAD) and nicotinamide adenine dinulceotide phosphate (NADP), that has to be supplied by the diet. In addition the amino acid, tryptophan, has a minor metabolic pathway via kynurenine to nicotinate; about 1/60 of ingested tryptophan goes this way. Tryptophan makes up about 1% of dietary proteins, so 70 g protein a day provides about 12 mg niacin equivalents towards the total niacin requirement of 15–18 mg a day (for adults).

Pellagra, caused by niacin deficiency, is now rare except in areas, such as parts of Africa, where people subsist on maize and little else. The niacin in maize is in a bound form, biologically unavailable (except when cooked the Central American way), and tryptophan is its limiting amino acid (unlike other cereals). Secondary pellagra may occur in patients with chronic renal failure on low protein diets or dialysis if niacin is not included in the regimen. Another rare cause is Hartnup disease, a recessive inborn error of tryptophan absorption first reported from the Middlesex Hospital, London.

Above the nutrient dose nicotinic acid produces cutaneous flushing from histamine release at doses of 100 mg/day or more; it has been used for chilblains. At doses 3 g/day or more it inhibits lipolysis in adipose tissue and lowers plasma cholesterol and triglyceride concentrations. It is one of the standard treatments for combined hyperlipidaemia—that is, hypercholesterolaemia plus hypertriglyceridaemia. Patients often develop tolerance to the flushing. Its other side effects (in high dosage) include gastric irritation, hyperuricaemia, impaired glucose tolerance and liver function tests and occasionally cholestatic jaundice.

Vitamin B-6

The term vitamin B-6 includes five closely related substances that all occur in foods and in the body: pyridoxal and pyridoxamine, their 5' phosphates, and pyridoxine, best known to doctors as the pharmaceutical form. Primary dietary deficiency is rare. An outbreak of convulsions in infants in 1954 was traced to insufficient vitamin B-6 in milk formula because of a manufacturing error. Several drugs interfere with vitamin B-6: hydralazine, penicillamine, and possibly oestrogens. Peripheral neuropathy from high dose isoniazid is prevented with pyridoxine. There are several conditions for which pharmacological doses of 50 to 100 mg pyridoxine are probably beneficial. These include homocystinuria, hyperoxaluria, gyrate atrophy of the choroid, hypochromic sideroblastic anaemia, and radiation sickness. Some biochemical indices of vitamin B-6 state may be abnormal in women taking some oral contraceptives, but these are indirect indices. The more specific plasma pyridoxal phosphate concentration is usually normal. Premenstrual tension is a very variable condition: prescribed or self medication with pyridoxine has no physiological basis and has never been subjected to a convincing double blind trial.

Above 200 mg/day pyridoxine may cause severe sensory neuropathy.[1] All seven patients in the first report of this side effect were taking pyridoxine for an inadequate indication—mostly for premenstrual oedema—and most had increased the dosage on their own. Pyridoxine should not be available over the counter at tablet size above 50 mg (which is already 25 times the nutrient requirement).

Food sources of vitamin B-6

Liver

whole grain cereals,

meat, fish,

peanuts, bananas,

walnuts, avocados,

potatoes, beans

Vitamin B-12

The red vitamin was the last to be isolated (1948). Humans eat it preformed in animal foods including fish and milk. It is synthesised by some microorganisms—for example, in the rumen of cows and sheep (which require traces of cobalt in the pasture). No vegetable food has been shown to contain vitamin B-12 consistently unless it is contaminated—for example, by manure. Humans excrete in the faeces vitamin B-12 that has been synthesised by the colonic bacteria. Vitamin B-12 is the largest of the nutrients, with a molecular weight of about 1350. The physiological mechanism for its absorption requires intrinsic factor from the stomach, and the complex is absorbed only at a special site, in the terminal ileum. Deficiency occurs in several gastric, intestinal, and ileal diseases, incuding pernicious anaemia, and in vegans (pure vegetarians). Adult body stores of vitamin B-12 in the liver last longer than those for any other vitamin, but deficiency occurs more quickly in infants. Vitamin B-12 cooperates with folate in DNA synthesis, so deficiency of either leads to megaloblastosis. Vitamin B-12 has a separate biochemical role, unrelated to folate, in synthesising fatty acids in myelin, so deficiency can present with neurological symptoms. Deficiency is diagnosed by measuring the serum vitamin B-12 concentration.

Supplementation with hydroxocobalamin is desirable for adult vegans and essential for their young children. Several drugs, such as colchicine and metformin, and prolonged anaesthesia with nitrous oxide, can interfere with absorption of vitamin B-12. Hydroxocobalamin can improve some cases of optic neuritis, possibly by detoxifying accumulated cyanide. Apart from rare hypersensitivity reactions there are no known toxic effects from vitamin B-12. It thus makes an ideal placebo, which may still be the commonest reason for its prescription.

Food sources of vitamin B-12

Liver (richest source),

kidney,

sardines,

oysters,

heart,

rabbit,

other meats, fish,

eggs,

cheese,

milk

Folate

Folic acid (pteroylglutamic acid) is the primary vitamin from the chemical point of view, and this is the pharmaceutical form because of its stability. But it is rare in foods or in the body. Most folates are in the reduced form (tetrahydrofolate); they have one-carbon components attached, and up to seven (instead of one) glutamic acid residues. These folates have many essential roles in one-carbon transfers in the body, including one of the steps in DNA synthesis.

In folate deficiency there is first a reduction of serum folate below 3 ng/ml and later megaloblastosis of blood cells and other cells with a rapid turnover. As well as anaemia, diarrhoea is common when the deficiency results from antagonism (due to drugs) rather than dietary lack.

Folate deficiency may occur simply from a poor diet, but it is usually seen when there is malabsorption or increased requirements because of pregnancy (see chapter 4) or increased cell proliferation (haemopoiesis, lymphoproliferative disorders) or antagonism from a number of drugs. Methotrexate, aminopterin, pyrimethamine, and co-trimoxazole act by inhibiting the complete reduction of folate to the active form, tetrahydrofolate, preferentially in cancer cells or micro-organisms. Alcoholism is the commonest antagonist.

Body stores of folate are not large and deficiency can develop quickly in patients on intensive therapy. In some cases this can be ascribed to intravenous alcohol or particular parenteral amino acid mixtures. Trauma, infection, uraemia, increased haemopoiesis, dialysis, vomiting, or diarrhoea may also be partly responsible. Folate deficiency appears to be the most common vitamin deficiency among adult hospital patients in countries such as Britain, so supplements should be prescribed whenever patients are fed intravenously for more than a few days.

The name comes from the Latin *folia* (= leaf), but liver, legumes, nuts, and even wholemeal bread are as good dietary sources as leafy vegetables. Prolonged boiling destroys much of the vitamin in hospital cabbage. No serious toxic effects are known from moderate doses (large doses cannot be bought over the counter) except the possibility of masking vitamin B-12 deficiency: anaemia is corrected but spinal cord lesions (subacute combined degeneration) get worse. For this reason multivitamin preparations do not usually contain folic acid (Pregnavite Forte F is an exception—see chapter 4).

Food sources of folate

Liver,

kidney, spinach,

broccoli,

Lima beans, beetroot,

bran,

peanuts,

cabbage, lettuce,

avocados, bananas,

oranges,

wholemeal bread,

eggs,

some fish

In Britain total vegetables provide 35%, bread and flour products 26%, fruit 6%

Vitamin C

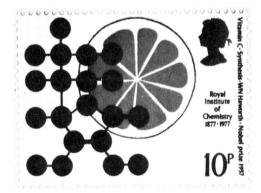

Ascorbic acid is the major antioxidant in the aqueous phase of the body. The best established biochemical consequence of its deficiency is imparied reduction of the amino acid, proline, to hydroxyproline. Hydroxyproline is an uncommon amino acid, except in collagen, of which it makes up an indispensable 12%. Impaired collagen formation is the biochemical basis of scurvy.

Small doses of vitamin C will cure scurvy. Lind achieved this with two oranges and a lemon in the first controlled trial on HMS *Salisbury* in 1747 (see back cover); 30 mg of vitamin C is more than enough to prevent scurvy.

Desirable intakes of vitamin C can be thought of at three levels.
(1) The official recommended intake for adults—30 mg/day in Britain and 60 mg/day in the USA and Canada—is for healthy people.
(2) In hospital patients this is not enough. Absorption of the vitamin may be reduced or its catabolism increased by disease. Trauma and surgery increase the need for vitamin C for collagen synthesis. Several drugs antagonise vitamin C: adrenal corticosteroids, aspirin, indomethacin, phenylbutazone, and tetracycline, together with smoking. Hence it is advisable to give a supplement of up to 250 mg ascorbic acid a day to cover major surgery.
(3) The third level is the great vitamin C debate: megadoses (up to 10 g/day) proposed by Linus Pauling for superhealth—or not? The best known claim for large intakes of vitamin C is that they prevent common colds. At least 31 controlled trials have been reported and in 23 of them (including the largest and best designed ones) there was no significant preventive effect. The eight supportive trials all had qualifications—for example, they were not double blind, had tiny groups, or showed an effect only in a subgroup.[2] At high dosage most of the vitamin does not appear to be absorbed. The law of diminishing returns applies. Large intakes of vitamin C have several disadvantages. They produce moderate increases in urinary oxalate and urate excretions, which are undesirable in people with a tendency to form kidney stones, as well as dyspepsia and diarrhoea.

Food sources of vitamin C

Blackcurrants, guavas,

rosehip syrup, green peppers,

oranges, other citrus fruit, strawberries,

cauliflower, broccoli,

sprouts, cabbage, watercress,

potatoes,

(liver and milk)

In Britain on average vegetables supply 48% (21% from potatoes) and fruits contribute 41%

Vitamins

Vitamin D

7-dehydrocholesterol

↓ UV light (290-312 nm)

Cholecalciferol, vitamin D_3

(in the liver) ↓

25-hydroxycholecalciferol

(in kidneys) ↓

1,25-dihydroxycholecalciferol (calcitriol)

Food sources of vitamin D

Fish liver oils,

fatty fish (sardines,

herring, mackerel, tuna,

salmon, pilchards),

margarine (fortified),

infant milk formulas (fortified),

eggs, liver

In Britain on average margarine supplies 44%

Vitamin E

Food sources of vitamin E

Vegetable oils – wheat germ oil the richest,

margarines,

eggs, butter,

wholemeal cereals,

broccoli

Nevertheless, two gastrointestinal actions of vitamin C make it desirable for people to eat more than the basic recommended dietary intake of 30 mg. It enhances iron absorption from vegetable foods and it inhibits nitrosamine formation. The latter may explain the negative epidemiological associations between vitamin C intake and gastric cancer.

Vitamin C is easily destroyed by cooking (aggravated by alkaline conditions), so fresh fruit and salads should be encouraged and vegetables cooked lightly and quickly.

Cholecalciferol is hydroxylated in the liver to 25-OHD_3, the plasma concentration of which is a good index of vitamin D status. In the kidney 25-OHD_3 is further hydroxylated either to $1,25(OH_2)D_3$ (calcitriol) or to an inactive metabolite. Calcitriol functions as a hormone whose best known action is to stimulate the synthesis of a calcium transport protein in the epithelium of the small intestines.

The natural substance cholecalciferol was originally called vitamin D_3. Vitamin D_2 is the artificially produced ergocalciferol. The natural and usual source of cholecalciferol is by the action of short wavelength ultraviolet light from the sun on a companion of cholesterol in the skin, 7-dehydrocholesterol. Cholecalciferol also occurs in a small minority of our foods. When people live in high latitudes, wear clothes, and spend nearly all the time indoors and the sky is polluted with smoke they have insufficient exposure to ultraviolet light to make the required amount of this substance; under these conditions dietary intake becomes critical and cholecalciferol assumes the role of a vitamin.

In rickets and osteomalacia there is reduced calcification of growing and mature bones respectively. These diseases appear to be more prevalent in the United Kingdom than in other Western countries. They tend to affect adolescents and the elderly, especially Asians in northern cities. In Britons with normal levels plasma 25-OHD_3 concentrations show annual fluctuations, with their trough in late winter and their peak after the summer holidays. It is not clear whether the lower prevalence of rickets in Canada and Sweden is because milk is fortified with vitamin D or because people receive more ultraviolet radiation of their skin over the year in those other northern countries.

The small dietary contribution of vitamin D is lost in malabsorption and chronic biliary obstruction. Long term anticonvulsants, phenobarbitone and phenytoin, increase metabolic losses. Vitamin D is indicated in these conditions. In chronic renal failure and hypoparathyroidism $1\,\alpha$-hydroxylation to the active metabolite is impaired and the bone disease responds only to $1,25(OH)_2D_3$(calcitriol) or $1\,\alpha$-OHD_3 (alfacalcidol), a synthetic derivative.

Irradiation of the skin may cause sunburn but does not lead to vitamin D toxicity. On the other hand, the margin of safety with oral vitamin D, between the nutrient requirements of up to 10 µg and toxic intakes, is narrow. Overdose with vitamin D causes hypercalcaemia, with thirst, anorexia, polyuria, and the risk of metastatic calcification. Some children have developed hypercalcaemia on vitamin D intakes only five times the recommended nutrient intake. More than this should not be taken except for rickets or osteomalacia. Here 25 to 100 µg vitamin D—for example, as ergocalciferol—is the usual therapeutic dose.

[One international unit (IU, obsolescent) of vitamin D = 0·025 µg of cholecalciferol or ergocalciferol—that is, to convert IU to micrograms, divide by 40.]

Alpha tocopherol is the most active of eight very similar compounds with vitamin E activity. Being fat soluble, vitamin E is present in all cell membranes, where it is thought to reduce peroxidation of unsaturated fatty acids by free oxygen radicals.

The nutritional requirement for vitamin E is roughly proportional to the intake of polyunsaturated fat. Vitamin E is not easily transported across the placenta, and signs of deficiency are sometimes found in premature infants.

Four members of the vitamin E family are α-, β-, γ-, and δ-*tocopherol*. These differ chemically in the number and position of methyl groups on the double ring at one end of the molecule. Biologically α-tocopherol is the most potent and β, γ, and δ are each in turn less active. The tocopherols are more active than the four *tocotrienols*, which have double bonds in the side chain; α-tocotrienol is the most biopotent, next β-tocotrienol.

The eight vitamin E compounds also show d- and l- stereoisomerism. Natural forms are d- (or RRR) and synthetic are dl- (or racemic). Both forms of α-tocopherol are available commercially. The most biogiclly active compound is the natural d- (or RRR) α-tocopherol, and vitamin E activity in foods or tissues is summed as d- (or RRR) α-tocopherol equivalents.

Patients with deficiency have a mild haemolytic anaemia, low plasma tocopherol concentration, and red cells abnormally sensitive to haemolysis in vitro by dilute hydrogen peroxide. The most severe cases of deficiency occur in patients with fat malabsorption, especially fibrocystic disease of the pancreas and abetalipoproteinaemia. As well as mild anaemia, in these conditions ataxia, loss of tendon jerks, and pigmentary retinopathy have been reported, which respond to long term vitamin E treatment.

Doses of vitamin E above the recommended 10 mg/day reduce the severity of retrolental fibroplasia in premature newborn infants who require oxygen. Many people now take vitamin E in large doses on their own initiative. In a double blind trial this showed no benefits on work performance, sexuality, or general well being. It is also clear from several trials that vitamin E does not improve athletic achievement or consistently help angina pectoris. Although it is a fat soluble vitamin, tocopherol, however, seems to have low toxicity.

Vitamin K

Food sources of vitamin K

Turnip greens,

broccoli,

cabbage, lettuce,

liver,

are all good sources, though there is no

systematic list

The Koagulations vitamin (Dam, 1935) comes in three chemical forms. Vitamin K_1 (phytomenadione) is found mainly in vegetables. The series of K_2 vitamins (menaquinones) is produced by bacteria—for example, in the gut. Menadione (Synkavit) is synthetic, water soluble, can cause jaundice, and is obsolescent. Deficiency of vitamin K manifests itself as hypoprothrombinaemia and bleeding.

Cord blood levels of vitamin K are very low (evidently placental transfer is limited), and breast milk contains little of the vitamin unless the mother has been dosed with vitamin K. To prevent haemorrhagic disease of the newborn 1 mg of vitamin K_1 (by injection or by mouth) is given either to all infants or to those at increased risk (low birth weight or difficult delivery), depending on the hospital's policy.

In adults vitamin K deficiency is to be expected in obstructive jaundice and can occur in malabsorption syndromes. Vitamin K_1 must be given before surgery for these conditions. Anticoagulants of the warfarin group owe their thereapeutic action to antagonism of vitamin K, and vitamin K_1 is the antidote to overdose.

Vitamins that can usually be taken for granted

Not vitamins

The following compounds sold in "health

food" shops and still included in some

multivitamin pharmaceuticals are not vitamins.

They are not required in infant formulas or in

fluids for total parenteral nutrition:

Bioflavinoids

Inositol

Orotic acid

Aminobenzoic acid (PABA)

Vitamin B15 ("pangamic acid")

Vitamin B17 (laetrile)

Vitamin P

Biotin is cofactor for several carboxylase enzymes concerned in fat synthesis and amino acid catabolism. It is widely distributed in foods, the requirement is small, and deficiency is rare. Deficiency has occurred in people who eat large amounts of raw eggs (which contain a protein that binds biotin and prevents its absorption) and in patients receiving total parenteral nutrition with biotin omitted. They suffer scaly dermatitis, loss of hair, hypercholesterolaemia, and a characteristic combination of organic acids in the urine.

Pantothenic acid is a constituent of coenzyme A which has many functions and is widespread in the body and in foods. The name means "available everywhere." Spontaneous deficiency in man has never been proved.

Choline is part of lecithin and of sphingomyelin, the two major phospholipids in the body, and it is also part of acetylcholine, the neutrotransmitter. It is a dietary essential for the rat, but man seems to be able to synthesise it (partly from methionine) and does not have the active catabolising enzyme (choline oxidase) found in rat liver. Pharmacological doses as choline or lecithin are being used to treat tardive dyskinesia and some other neurological disorders. Depression is a side effect.

1 Parry GJ, Bredesden DE. Sensory neuropathy with low-dose pyridoxine. *Neurology* 1985;35:1466–8.
2 Truswell AS. Ascorbic acid and colds. *N Engl J Med* 1986; 315: 709.

11: OBESITY

Diagnosis and risks

In 1987 in Great Britain 8% of men and 12% of women aged 16–64 were obese (weight/height$^2 \geqslant 30$)[1]

   10% of 36 million people = 3·6 million obese people

   In 1989 there were 1408 wte (whole time equivalent) dietitians and 30 631 general practitioner principals

   Thus 1 dietitian to every 2557 obese people and 117 obese people for every GP principal

NHS consultants in England, 1989

Cardiologists	144
General surgeons	943
Ophthalmologists	450
Rheumatologists	234
Obesity specialists	1 (? more)

It is easy to diagnose moderate and gross obesity before the patient undresses. The difficulty with these patients is to organise the time and summon up the enthusiasm to embark on treatment which will be lengthy and may be unsuccessful. When our profession can transplant a human heart, manage in vitro fertilisation, and eliminate smallpox, to treat obesity is a challenge for a conscientious practitioner. A health service, like the British NHS, which provides an annual fee per patient is a suitable framework.

Obesity is different from most other serious diseases. If the general practitioner feels he is not the best person to look after a patient's haemorrhoids or backache or poor vision there is usually a specialist at the nearest big hospital who has the skills and equipment and will be happy to manage this part of the patient. But there is unlikely to be a consultant with special skills or equipment for looking after obesity.

Many obese patients are referred to dietitians but there are too many obese people for the number of dietitians in Britain, and hospital staff are not well placed for looking after obese "outpatients"—that is, people who live at home and have to go out to work each weekday.

To put in the hard work of treating the obese people on the practice's list reduces the likelihood of having to treat them later for complications of obesity.

Managing obesity: the advantages of general practice

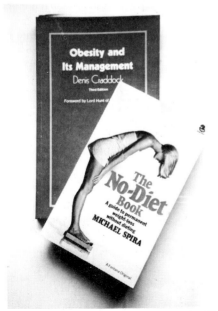

The best conditions for managing obesity are:

- Regular visits, at least once a fortnight
- Weighing the patient under the same conditions on the same scale
- About 1/4 hour talk with the same practitioner each visit
- Opportunity to bring wife or husband
- The therapist is not obese.

The first four conditions are easier for the patient in general practice.

Two general practitioners' books about their work with obese patients

Complications of obesity

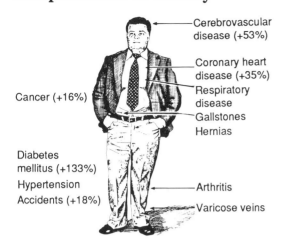

Obesity increases the risk of mortality from some of these diseases (notably diabetes) more than others

"Make less thy body hence, and more thy grace;
Leave gormandising; know the grave doth gape
For thee thrice wider than for other men."
SHAKESPEARE, *King Henry IV* Part II, V, v.

Most of the medical complications of obesity are well known. Risks of cardiovascular complications and diabetes are greater in people with abdominal obesity, that is, with an increased waist/hip circumference ratio (waist measured at the umbilicus, hip at the maximum protuberance of the buttocks).[2] The ratio should not exceed 0·85 for men and 0·75 for women under 40 and 0·95 for men and 0·8 for women thereafter. Considerable weight gain in a short time carries greater risks than reaching the same weight slowly.[3]

The social complications are more immediate and may be very painful. Religious, racial, and gender prejudice are now unacceptable in mainstream Western societies, as is prejudice against the disabled. But prejudice against fat people is undisguised. It starts at school, affects the job opportunities and social status of obese people—and it is so pervasive that it probably colours many doctors' attitudes towards their obese patients.

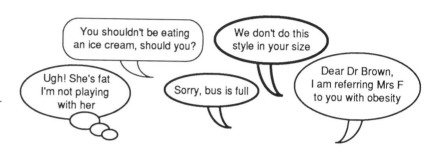

Mild obesity

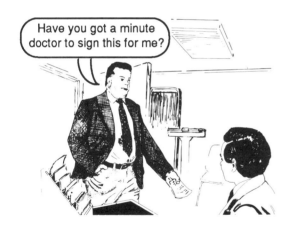

By contrast, for mild obesity diagnosis and recognition are where the management goes wrong. Yet there are several people with mild obesity for every case of obvious obesity in a practice. Mild obesity is much easier to treat, and prevention of gross obesity is much easier than cure.

People with mild obesity do not usually come to their practitioner complaining that they are too fat. The adiposity has been slowly creeping up on them and does not cause pain, distress, or fear. They present with any other symptom and disease.

Patients may become mildly obese under their doctor's eyes, during the course of an illness which the practitioner is following and concentrating on: bed rest after myocardial infarction; giving up smoking; pregnancy and lactation; anxiety or depression from stress at work or at home. Recognition of mild obesity can be more difficult too in a patient in bed.

"No woman can be too thin or too rich"

—DUCHESS OF WINDSOR

Measuring obesity

Measuring the patient

- Beam and lever scales are more reliable but take more space and are slower to use.

- For screening it is a good idea to have a lever scale in the reception area and for the receptionist or nurse to weigh the patient with shoes and coat removed.

- Obese patients being treated can be weighed (ideally in their underclothes) at each visit by the doctor in his consulting room on the same platform scale with a quick reading dial.

- The patient's height can be measured with a rule or tape measure attached to a flat wall and recorded in the notes. Heights are lower in the evening than in the morning. If the patient has any weakness or deformity an assistant is needed to get him as straight as possible for the measurement.

It is part of good practice to have a system so that all patients on the list are weighed at regular intervals by the receptionist or nurse. The weight is entered on the record. Knowing the patient's height (without shoes) the doctor can then decide whether he or she is: underweight, in the normal range, mildly overweight, or obese. Comparison with previous weights shows if the patient is putting on weight.

Weight measurements are objective. To show the patient his or her weight against the standards for his or her height is impressive and, if outside the normal range, the basis for action.

Obesity

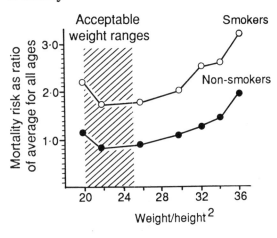

Acceptable weight ranges

Smokers

Non-smokers

Mortality risk as ratio of average for all ages

Weight/height²

Obesity is an excess of adipose tissue. There are two methods for deciding whether someone is too fat. One is social or according to fashion. The doctor's role here is to advise patients not to make themselves too thin, not to take unphysiological diets or drugs to lose weight unnecessarily, and not to start on the road to anorexia nervosa.

The other method for deciding whether someone is too fat (or too thin) is actuarial. Above (or below) a range of weights for a given height the risk of developing illness or of mortality increases. Weight/height² (in kg/m²) is a convenient index of relative weight. It gives a single number and is almost independent of height. It is also called the body mass index (BMI) or Quetelet's index. Note that smoking carries a higher risk of mortality than overweight or the milder degrees of obesity.

Variations in mortality by weight among 750 000 men and women.[4]

Guidelines for body weight in adults

Height without shoes		Weight (kg) without clothes		
m	feet, inches	Acceptable	Obese	(Grossly obese)
1·45	4,9	42–53	64	(85)
1·48	4,10	42–54	65	(86)
1·50	4,11	43–55	66	(88)
1·52	5,0	44–57	68	(90)
1·54	5,1	44–58	70	(93)
1·56	5,1	45–58	70	(93)
1·58	5,2	51–64	77	(102)
1·60	5,3	52–65	78	(104)
1·62	5,4	53–66	79	(105)
1·64	5,5	54–67	80	(106)
1·66	5,5	55–69	83	(110)
1·68	5,6	56–71	85	(113)
1·70	5,7	58–73	88	(117)
1·72	5,8	59–74	89	(118)
1·74	5,9	60–75	90	(120)
1·76	5,9	62–77	92	(122)
1·78	5,10	64–79	95	(126)
1·80	5,11	65–80	96	(128)
1·82	6,0	66–82	98	(130)
1·84	6,0	67–84	101	(134)
1·86	6,1	69–86	103	(137)
1·88	6,2	71–88	106	(141)
1·90	6,3	73–90	108	(144)
1·92	6,4	75–93	112	(150)

Acceptable weights are W/H² 20–25.
Obesity is taken to start at W/H² 30 and gross obesity at W/H² 40.
[Partly based on table I from Royal College of Physician's report *Obesity*, 1983,[5] and Garrow *Treat Obesity Seriously*, 1981.[6]]
Patients between acceptable weight and obese are "overweight" (eg 75–90 kg if 1·74 m tall)

There are other standards but most are similar or related. The lower and upper ends of the acceptable range here are close to, respectively, the lowest weight for small frame and highest weight for large frame for men in the "desirable weights" of the Metropolitan Life Insurance Company of New York (1959).

The unisex table given here is a new practice: older standards had somewhat lower cut off points for women than men, but the numbers of women taking out life insurance were probably inadequate. Modern prospective data show no significant differences between men and women.

Obesity is taken in this table and generally as starting at 20% above the upper end of the acceptable range of weights. Grades of obesity can thus be expressed: 20% above acceptable, 30% above, 40%, etc. The figures in the grossly obese column are 60% above the upper acceptable figure. Men of this weight have at least 200% the mortality of people with normal ("acceptable") weight.

The cut off values in the table have to be read from the viewpoint of the individual patient, like normal ranges for laboratory tests. People with gracile bones should weigh less than heavy boned people. Unusual muscle development (as in weight lifters) and oedema increase body weight. The waist/hip ratio should also be included in the assessment.

Suggested cut offs for overweight children

Age (years)	Boys		Girls	
	Average height (cm)	97th percentile weight (kg) for average height	Average height (cm)	97th percentile weight (kg) for average height
2·0	86	14·9	84	14·2
2·5	90	16·9	90	15·3
3·0	95	17·3	94	16·8
3·5	99	18·5	98	18·0
4·0	103	19·7	102	19·0
4·5	107	20·8	105	20·1
5·0	110	22·0	108	21·3
5·5	113	23·2	112	22·4
6·0	116	24·6	115	23·7
6·5	119	26·1	118	25·2
7·0	122	27·5	121	27·0
7·5	124	29·5	123	28·6
8·0	127	31·2	126	31·4
8·5	130	33·1	129	34·1
9·0	132	35·2	132	36·7
9·5	135	37·8	135	40·3
10·0	138	40·2	—	—

In children there are no actuarial data on which to base cut off weights for obesity. However, the 97th percentile weight for age of the US National Center for Health Statistics standards can provide objective figures for overweight (used in the table). They need to be adjusted if the child is unusually short or tall.

For adolescents it is recommended that the start of obesity be taken at 20% above average weight for height. No single column of numbers can be given for this, however, because of the varying times of onset of puberty. A four-page table in the Royal College of Physicians "*Obesity*" report (1983) can be referred to.

Causes

Obesity *secondary* to hypothalamic conditions that increase appetite is rare and to endocrine disorders uncommon. It is not practical to send the large numbers of obese people throughout the country for expensive endocrinological investigations.

Obesity may follow (*a*) enforced inactivity such as bed rest, arthritis, stroke, change to a less active job, sports injury, or (*b*) overeating associated with psychological disturbances or some drugs that increase the appetite: adrenocortical steroids, sulphonylureas, anabolic agents, oral contraceptives, and cyproheptidine (Periactin).

The genetic influence on obesity was clearly shown in a study using the Danish Adoption Register. A strong relation existed between the weight class of the adoptees (thin, acceptable, overweight, or obese) and the body mass index of their biological, but not their adoptive, parents.[7] In Britain, body mass index is more strongly correlated between monozygotic than dizygotic twins, even when they are reared apart.[8]

In the great majority obesity is *primary*. There is no obvious predisposing condition. If the patient says she eats little: (1) The weight gain may have been in the past. (2) Some people undoubtedly need less food than others apparently comparable; they are efficient metabolisers with a low basal metabolic rate (but normal thyroid) and may feel the cold sooner than others. (3) Repeated periods on low calorie diets may lead to further adaptive lowering of the basal metabolic rate.

In surveys, obese people have often been found not to eat more than thin people. But the new doubly labelled water technique (that measures rates of disappearence of the stable isotopes, ^{2}H and ^{18}O) showed that the energy expenditure of a group of obese people was higher than their self recorded food energy intakes.[9]

No single mechanism has been consistently confirmed in all obese people —whether lack of brown adipose tissue, inactive sodium pumps, low basal metabolic rate, distored appetite regulation, less glycogen and more fat synthesis, fewer slow muscle fibres (which combust fatty acids), etc, etc.

Obesity is a syndrome, like fever or anaemia, with no single cause.

Management

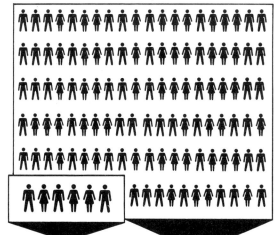

117 Patients per GP

Grossly obese—specialist management

111 Moderately obese —managed by GP

Management should fit the grade of the obesity.

Gross obesity is rare, and ideally such patients should be referred to a special centre. Surgery such as gastric stapling or jaw wiring may be justifiable. (The complications of ileal bypass are formidable.)

For patients with *moderate obesity* (W/H^2 30–39) regular repeated visits to general practitioners are justified and anorectic drugs if indicated. Aims should be realistic. The alternative is referral to slimming clubs, NHS dietitians, or commercial organisations with occasional checks by the general practitioner.

Principles of reducing regimen

> You can lose weight only by achieving a cumulative negative energy balance. Calories in must be less than calories expended. An average loss of 2000 kJ (500 kcal) per day—14 000 kJ (3500 kcal) over a week—is equivalent to a loss of about 0·5 kg (1 lb) per week or more at the start, when water is lost.

Some useful questions:

Why do you want to lose weight?
What weight would *you* like to be?
Are you on a diet now?
What diets have you been on before, and what happened?
Who shops and cooks at home?
What do your family think? Will they support you?

Alternative or supplementary strategies to close personal management

● Hand out a diet sheet. The most dismissive course and least recommended. The new eating regimen needs to be tailored to the individual patient.

● Recommend a popular book—such as the F plan diet or the Prudent diet. Others are often unphysiological and dangerous (see *BMJ* 1982;**285**:1519).

● Recommend a good local slimming club (eg Weight Watchers), group therapy.

● Refer the patient to a dietitian, preferably nearby and linked with the practice.

The essence of treatment is to reduce the food energy. Most people experience periods of hunger, all are deprived of their accustomed amount of oral gratification and suffer repeated temptations.

To stick to a weight-reducing diet is a battle of the will—the patient's own will. Motivation is essential. No patient will go day after day denying himself or herself the usual pleasures of eating unless he or she is motivated to persevere and can see rewards ahead such as better health or a more attractive appearance. Sometimes a fat patient is not ready to embark on a long and strenuous course of weight reduction on the day the doctor first broaches it. He or she may be going through a personal crisis, which is reflected in the obesity. If the doctor is understanding the fat person may later be able to follow the advice given below. Obese people can have low self esteem. The therapist needs to strengthen this and build up the patient's motivation.

● Habits are more important than diets.
● It is the long haul that counts.
● Crash diets and gimmicks do not work and may be dangerous.
● A loss of 2 kg per week for the first week and then 1 kg per week is as much as can be expected but half this is acceptable (and all that some can manage).

The nutritional principles are simple:

● Eat less—eat 2/3 or 1/2 the calories (joules) you have been eating.
● Technically the usual aim is about 4·2 MJ/day (1000 kcal/day) for a woman, 6·3 MJ/day (1500 kcal/day) for a man.
● Try to cut out empty calorie foods—fats, alcohol, and sugars, which provide 38, 29, and 16 kJ/g (9, 7, and 4 kcal/g) respectively—especially fats, as the homeostatic mechanisms that increase the oxidation of carbohydrate after its consumption do not exist for fats.[10]
● Eat three meals a day.
● Have a variety of foods each day from the major four food groups—meat and fish, milk and cheese, bread and cereals, vegetables and fruits.
● The amounts of low calorie foods (see table) can be maintained or even increased.
● Special dietary foods are unnecessary.
● Do not buy or keep in the house the food(s) that you find most tempting, "more-ish."
● A calorie counter can interest the patient who likes to go into details but carbohydrate counting is unphysiological.
● There is a considerable range of calorie values for typical servings of common foods (see table).
● Very low calorie diets (less than 2·5 MJ (600 kcal) a day) are likely to induce more loss of lean body mass (muscle, etc) than the gentler regimen above and have not been shown to be more effective in the long run. They are contraindicated in several conditions and should not be taken alone for more than 3–4 weeks.[11] Their administration is best left to specialists.

Representative energy values of stated typical servings of some common foods

	kJ	kcal		kJ	kcal		kJ	kcal
Lettuce (30 g)	17	4	Egg (1 boiled)	305	73	Peanuts (30 g)	711	170
Cucumber (45 g)	21	5	Banana (1 fruit)	334	80	Avocado ($\frac{1}{2}$ fruit)	711	170
Carrot (50 g)	42	10	Beer ($\frac{1}{2}$ pint)	360	86	Chicken (roast, meat only,		
Cauliflower (90 g, raw)	50	12	Wine (125 g)	393	94	120 g)	744	178
Tomato (90 g)	54	13	Yoghurt (carton, low fat)	418	100	Cheese (Cheddar, 45 g)	752	180
Grapefruit ($\frac{1}{2}$, no sugar)	75	18	Cornflakes (30 g)	460	110	Chocolate biscuits (2)	794	190
Milk (full cream, 30 g, in tea)	84	20	Butter (15 g)	460	110	Beef steak (grilled, 150 g)	1003	240
Sugar (1 level teaspoon)	84	20	Fish (cod, grilled, 120 g)	481	115	Potato crisps (50 g)	1108	265
Crispbread (10 g)	134	32	Potatoes (boiled, 150 g)	481	115	Rice (75 g, raw)	1129	270
Jam (15 g)	168	40	Carbonated soft drink (323 ml)	543	130	Macaroni (75 g, raw)	1170	280
Orange juice (120 g)	192	46	Dates (60 g)	585	140	Sponge cake (65 g)	1212	290
Apple (100 g)	192	46	Baked beans (240 g)	606	145	Fish (fried in batter, 120 g)	1338	320
Peas (90 g)	209	50	Milk chocolate (30 g)	648	155	Chips (fried, 180 g)	1902	455
Whisky (25 g)	234	56	Biscuits (2 digestive)	670	160	Pork chops (fried, including		
Bread (1 slice, 30 g)	280	67				fat, 210 g with bone)	2257	540

Time	Food	Taste rating	Amount	kcal	Where?	Who with?	Mood	Hunger	Associated activity	Why eaten?
4.45pm	Chocolate Cake	My weakness V. Good	3 slices	510	Kitchen	Children	Fed up	No	Giving children their tea	Irritated
5.00pm	Egg Sandwiches	Nothing Special	1½ sandwiches	200	Kitchen	Alone	OK	No	Clearing	by noise Leftovers
6.00pm	Gin & Tonic Peanuts	✓ ✓	1 Large ½ pkt (1oz)	14						
7.30pm	Supper: Lamb chop Sprouts Potatoes	OK	Medium							

The central technique for managing obesity is modification of eating behaviour. Its introduction by R B Stuart in 1967 changed the expectation of treatment from poor to fair and refinements are improving prospects further.

First the patient makes notes of everthing he or she eats for a week and where they were at the time, what they were doing, and how they felt. The calories can be worked out later. The therapist guides and encourages the patient to fill in the form in detail. In the process the patient discovers in what circumstances he or she eats most. The doctor discusses the completed form with the patient and suggests behaviour modifications. More often than not, obese people do not eat because they are hungry, but in response to external cues—boredom, anger, delicious taste, other people eating, food that would be wasted, etc. The patient can make arrangements to minimise these cues.

Rules for modifying eating behaviour

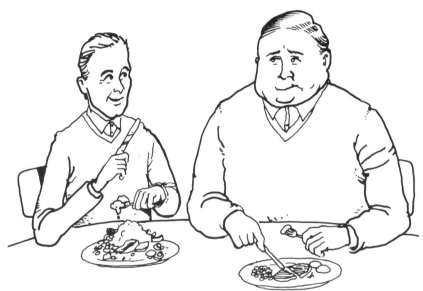

(1) Buy non-fattening foods. Do not buy foods that specially tempt you. Use a shopping list and stick to it. Do not shop when you are hungry.

(2) Always eat in one room, in only one place in that room—for example, seated at the dining table—and avoid other activities (except conversation). Make eating a pure experience.

(3) Look for times when you are most likely to eat unnecessarily—for example, when giving children their tea, or because you cannot bear to throw food away—and take steps to change your routine.

(4) Always have nearby a variety of low calorie foods to use as snacks—like raw vegetables.

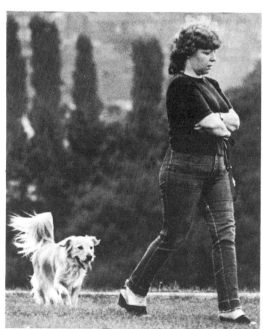

(5) Recruit others to help you curb your eating—spouse, coworkers, friends—they can help most by praising when you do not overeat.

(6) Build in rewards for sticking to the programme—sometimg you would like to do or a present. Family and friends are usually happy to cooperate. Of course, the reward cannot be a meal or food.

(7) Make small portions of food appear to be large (small plate, food cut up and spread all over it). Make second helpings hard to get; do not keep serving dishes on the table. Leave the table as soon as you have eaten.

(8) Slow down the rate at which you eat. Chew each mouthful for longer. Always use a knife and fork or a spoon and put them down between mouthfuls. Swallow one mouthful before the next.

(9) Take steps to minimise hunger, loneliness, depression, boredom, anger, and fatigue, each of which can set off a bout of overeating. This needs discussion and planning. Hunger is minimised by three regular meals daily.

(10) Increase the exercise you take each day.

(11) Keep a record of how much you eat and exercise and of your weight.

Obesity

Exercise

Energy/minute used in activities
(rounded approximate figures)

	kJ	kcal
At rest (Men + 10%, women − 10%)	4	1
Moderate exercise For example, walking, gardening, golf	21	5
Intermediate For example, cycling, swimming, tennis	29	7
Strenuous For example, squash, jogging, hill climbing, heavy work	42	10

In SI units: 1 kcal/min = 4·2 kJ/min = 70 watts

During an hour's walk at ordinary speed, mostly on the level, $21 \times 60 = 1260$ kJ ($5 \times 60 = 300$ kcal) of energy are used up. But at rest about $4·2 \times 60 = 252$ kJ ($1 \times 60 = 60$ kcal) would be spent per hour. The energy used by the effort of going for an hour's walk is therefore the difference between 1260 and 252 = 1008 kJ (300 and 60 = 240 kcal). This is equivalent to about two slices of bread and butter (60 g bread + 15 g butter, see table on previous page).

People can be discouraged by the small amount of food which is directly equivalent to the use of quite a lot of precious time taking exercise.

There are, however, additional benefits from increased regular exercise. Firstly, obese people, with a heavier body to move, use more energy for the same amount of work. Secondly, exercise can be valuable as a diversion from sitting indoors and being tempted to eat. Thirdly, exercise is more likely to reduce than increase appetite. Fourthly, after exercise the resting metabolic rate may increase for some hours (though the effect is evidently small, and some experimenters have not been able to measure it). Fifthly, when exercise is taken after meals the thermic effect of the meal may be increased.

Drugs

Diethylpropion, phentermine, and *chlorphentermine* are derivatives of amphetamines (controlled drugs which are subject, in the UK, to the prescription requirements of the Misuse of Drugs Regulations 1985). They reduce appetite by enhancing release of noradrenaline but are likely to cause some sleeplessness, nervousness, irritability, dry mouth, palpitations, and increase of blood pressure. Best taken before time of day when hunger is expected.

Dexfenfluramine is the D- (dextro-) isomer of the racemic mixture, D- and L-fenfluramine which was the older drug fenfluramine hydrochloride (Ponderax). It potentiates serotonin in the brain, and this increases satiety. Side effects include drowsiness, dry mouth, and diarrhoea. The dose is 15 mg twice a day at meal times; the course should not exceed three months. (Interactions can occur with appetite suppressants, also some antihypertensive, antidiabetic, sedative, and antidepressant drugs).

Anorectic drugs at present available are an optional extra to support behaviour modification and diet in some patients with moderate or gross obesity, particularly those who are persistently troubled by hunger on a reduced food intake. They are not justifiable for mildly overweight people because they have side effects, occasionally severe.

Diethylpropion (Tenuate) and phentermine (Preludin) are examples of the group that reduces appetite, but they tend to be sympathomimetic stimulants. They can be useful in a depressed obese patient and, being short acting, can be taken intermittently.

Dexfenfluramine and related drugs work in a different way: they increase satiety and take days for their effects to develop. It is reported that dexfenfluramine especially reduces intake of carbohydrate snacks, which often also contain fat. A steady reduction of dosage over one or two weeks is advisable because rapid withdrawal can be followed by depression.

1 Gregory J, Foster K, Tyler H, Wiseman M. *The dietary and nutritional survey of British adults*. London: HMSO, 1990.
2 Ashwell M, Cole TJ, Dixon AK. Obesity: new insight into the anthropometric classification of fat distribution shown by computed tomography. *BMJ* 1985;**290**:1692–4.
3 Wannamethee G, Shaper AG. Weight change in middle-aged British men: implications for health. *European Journal of Clinical Nutrition* 1990;**44**:133–42.
4 Lew EA, Garfinkel L. Variations in mortality by weight among 750 000 men and women. *Journal of Chronic Diseases* 1979;**32**:563–76.
5 Royal College of Physicians. Obesity. A report of the Royal College of Physicians. *J R Coll Physicians Lond* 1983;**17**:3–58.
6 Garrow JS. *Treat obesity seriously. A clinical manual*. Edinburgh and London: Churchill Livingstone, 1981.
7 Stunkard AJ, Sorensen TIA, Harris C, *et al*. An adoption study of human obesity. *N Engl J Med* 1986;**314**: 193–8.
8 Macdonald A, Stunkard A. Body-mass indexes of British separated twins. *N Engl J Med* 1990;**322**:1530.
9 Prentice AM, Black AE, Coward WA. High levels of energy expenditure in obese women. *BMJ* 1986;**292**:483–7.
10 Schutz Y, Jéquier E. Failure of dietary fat intake to promote fat oxidation: a factor favoring the development of obesity. *Am J Clin Nutr* 1989;**50**: 307–14.
11 Committee on Medical Aspects of Food Policy, Department of Health and Social Security. *The use of very low calorie diets in obesity*. London: HMSO, 1987. (Report on Health and Social Subjects No 31.)

12: MEASURING NUTRITION

Energy (calories)

The *nutritional state* for energy or for any essential nutrient depends on the balance (B) between intake (I) (dietary or parenteral) and output (O) or expenditure: B = I − O.

When the balance is negative the nutritional state tends to go down towards depletion, but there may be an adaptive reduction in output (losses). When the balance is positive the nutritional state tends to go up: the nutrient may be stored somewhere in the body but some nutrients can start to become toxic. "You can have too much of a good thing."

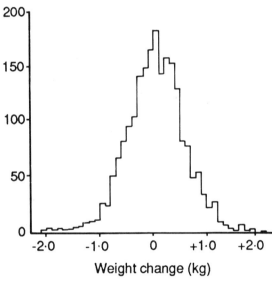

Distribution of day to day weight change (kg) on 2078 occasions on consecutive days in healthy young men[4]

Weight measurement

Beam or lever balances are most reliable, not the usual bathroom scales. The best scales are not easily portable: they are heavy and the knife edge balancing part can be damaged. The patient should if possible be brought to the scale. It should be serviced regularly (as recommended by the manufacturer) and checked frequently against known weights, such as a heavy weight kept nearby. Subjects should be weighed in light underclothing and no shoes and with any heavy jewellery removed. A meal or full bladder increases the reading and a bowel action reduces it.

Adults and older children should stand straight on both feet on the centre of the scale's platform without touching anything else.

Pictures of how to weigh young children are shown in Valman H B. *The First Year of Life*. 3rd ed. London: BMJ, 1989:91.

Methods of measuring calories (food energy) are different from those for the other essential nutrients.

Measurement of energy balance is technically difficult. **Energy expenditure** can be measured in one of six ways:

(1) By measuring a subject's heat output in a special insulated room. This is *direct calorimetry*, a costly and complicated experiment. There are very few direct calorimeter rooms anywhere in the world. The method has been replaced by:

(2) *Indirect calorimetry* measures oxygen consumption and the production of carbon dioxide and urinary nitrogen. From these the mixture of carbohydrate, fat (exogenous or endogenous), and protein metabolised can be calculated. Heat production differs with the metabolic fuel (greater when fat is oxidised). These measurements can be made in a respiration chamber, in which a subject can live for a day or more and carry out various activities.[1]

(3) The energy equivalent of oxygen consumed happens to be much the same whichever of the three macronutrients is oxidised. Oxygen consumption is measured in a ventilated hood or a Benedict-Roth apparatus, and such apparatus is used clinically to measure resting or *basal metabolic rate*, which can be increased in patients—eg, after burns or trauma or with infections.

(4) The *doubly labelled water* method measures the decay of body water concentrations of the stable isotopes ^{2}H and ^{18}O. It is a new method, suitable for measuring total energy expenditure over 7–10 days, and depends on the principle that labelled oxygen is lost partly as carbon dioxide and partly as water and the rate of water loss is given by the decay of labelled hydrogen.[2] Unfortunately the heavy oxygen is very expensive.

(5) It ought to be possible to assess energy expenditure from an estimate of basal metabolic rate (from the patient's age, sex, and weight) and from recording all his activities (lying, sitting, walking upstairs, etc) throughout the day. Energy values for the different activities have to be assumed from reported values. The method is tedious and inaccurate.

(6) The possibilities for estimating energy expenditure are better by counting the heart rate for a day or more with a small portable cardiac monitor.[3]

On the intake side the energy (calorie) content of foods eaten should ideally be analysed chemically by measuring the protein, available carbohydrate, fat, and alcohol contents and multiplying each of these by their metabolisable energy values. Energy values in food tables are only estimated averages.

The usual way of estimating energy balance is, of course, from the resultant changes in body weight. A gain or loss of energy by the body of about 25–29 MJ (6000–7000 kcal) should, respectively, increase or reduce the weight by 1·0 kg. Most of this weight change is in fat, with a variable amount of water and a minority of muscle. Gain or loss of tissue needs to be over 1 kg to be detectable because, even with accurate weighing and on a constant regimen, healthy people's weights fluctuate within the day and from day to day. Furthermore, many scales and weighing techniques are not accurate.

Measuring nutrition

Reference standards for mid-arm circumference (mm)*

Age	MEN			WOMEN		
	50th	10th	5th	50th	10th	5th
		Centiles			Centiles	
19–24	308	272	262	265	230	221
25–34	319	282	271	277	240	233
35–44	326	287	278	290	251	241
45–54	322	281	267	299	256	242
55–64	317	273	258	303	254	243
65–74	307	263	248	299	252	240

Reference standards for triceps skinfold thickness (mm)*

Age	MEN			WOMEN		
	50th	10th	5th	50th	10th	5th
		Centiles			Centiles	
18–24	9·5	5	4	18	11·5	10
25–34	12	6	4·5	21	12	10
35–44	12	6	5	23	14	12
45–54	12	6	6	25	16	12
55–64	11	6	5	25	16	12
65–74	11	6	4	24	14	12

* Figures based on a large sample of healthy US citizens from Frisancho A R[5] and Bishop C W, et al.[6]

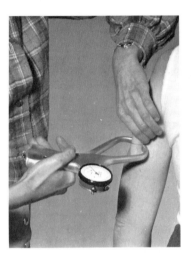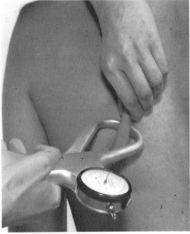

Measuring skinfold thickness with Holtain calipers: left—triceps site; right—subscapular site

Estimated average requirements of food energy for people in the United Kingdom[7]

Age	Males MJ/d (kcal/d)	Females MJ/d (kcal/d)
0–3 months	2·28 (545)	2·16 (515)
4–6 months	2·89 (690)	2·69 (645)
7–9 months	3·44 (825)	3·20 (765)
10–12 months	3·85 (920)	3·61 (865)
1–3 years	5·15 (1230)	4·86 (1165)
4–6 years	7·16 (1715)	6·46 (1545)
7–10 years	8·24 (1970)	7·28 (1740)
11–14 years	9·27 (2220)	7·92 (1845)
15–18 years	11·51 (2755)	8·83 (2110)
19–59 years	**10·60 (2550)**	**8·05 (1920)**
60–74 years	9·82 (2355)	7·98 (1900)
75 + years	8·77 (2100)	7·61 (1810)

Values from 0 to 18 years are based on average energy intakes. From 19 years on, however, they are based on measured energy expenditure, assuming low physical activity levels at work and leisure (physical activity level = 1·4 × BMR (basal metabolic rate)). More active people need to consume more than the figures here.

Reference standards for body weights at different heights are given for adults in chapter 11 (Obesity).

It is difficult to weigh deformed or paralysed people. Very sick bedfast people cannot be weighed unless they are in a specially designed weighing bed. It is nearly always easy to weigh an ambulant patient—it just takes a little time and trouble. But in hospital patients confined to bed—for example, those with fluid lines or splints—some idea of loss of tissue can be obtained by measuring the arm circumference with or without one or more skinfold thicknesses.

Measuring arm circumference needs only a tape measure, put round the arm (preferably left) midway between the tip of the acromion and the olecranon. The enclosed area is made up of muscles and subcutaneous fat over the constant humerus.

Measuring skinfold thickness requires special calipers. The best are obtainable from Holtain Ltd, Crymych, Dyfed SA41 3UF. Cheap plastic ones are unreliable. The most common sites for measuring skinfold thickness are over the mid-triceps, halfway between the acromion and the olecranon, and the subscapular skinfold, 1 cm below the inferior angle of the scapula. Reference standards are available for skinfolds at these sites.

The triceps skinfold measurement can be used to calculate the mid-arm muscle circumference, which is calculated as:

$$\text{arm circumference} - \pi \times \text{triceps skinfold (mm)}$$

Before substantial weight changes are detectable or if weight cannot be measured a rough idea of energy balance can be got by calculating the energy per day in recent food intake from food tables and comparing this with the estimated average requirements for energy published by the DoH.[7]

These reference values for energy intake are estimates and averages. They differ with gender, age, body weight, and activity level.[7] About half of any group of similar people can be expected to need more and half to need less than these values. Individual requirements might well range from 50% to 150% of these averages. Furthermore, on any single day an individual might consume considerably less or more than his average daily intake.

There are no biochemical tests that reliably indicate energy balance. Acetone appears on the breath in people who fast for longer than 12 hours and β hydroxybutyrate concentrations increase in body fluids but these cannot be used to show the extent of energy deficit.

Protein

Reference nutrient intake for protein,* based on British dietary reference values[7]

Age and sex	Body weight (kg)	Protein (g/kg body weight)	Reference nutrient intake (RNI) (g/day)
0–3 months	5·9	—	13
4–6 months	7·7	1·7	13
7–9 months	8·8	1·6	14
10–12 months	9·7	1·55	15
1–3 years	12·5	1·2	15
4–6 years	17·8	1·1	20
7–10 years	28·3	1·0	28
Males:			
11–14 years	43·0	1·0	43
15–18 years	64·5	0·86	55
19–50 years	74·0	0·75	56
50+ years	71·0	0·75	53
Females:			
11–14 years	43·8	1·0	44
15–18 years	55·5	0·81	45
19–50 years	60·0	0·75	45
50+ years	62·0	0·75	46
Pregnancy			+6
Lactation			+11

British dietary reference values are based on FAO/WHO (1984) safe levels of protein intake.
* These recommended intakes assume that the protein comes from a mixed diet, as in the average British diet. Requirements may be higher if digestibility of the protein is incomplete or if one (or more) of the indispensible amino acids is poorly represented.

Other nutrients

Check list on patient's diet

In a busy practice a short check list about the patient's eating habits is a useful screening method.

- What is your appetite like?
- Do you eat more or less than other comparable people?
- Has what you eat changed—type of food or amount?
- Are you on a special diet?
- Is there any food you can't eat because it doesn't agree with you?
- Are you losing or gaining body weight?
- What do you usually have for the main meal of the day?
- Do you eat meat/fruit/fat on meat/salt/etc?
- What sort of bread do you eat?
- What sort of alcohol do you drink, how many drinks per week or per day?
- What do you have for breakfast and lunch?
- Do you take vitamin or mineral tablets?

Tests for protein status estimate two variables: total body protein and visceral protein.

Total body protein (predominantly muscle) can be estimated in several ways, though the first two below are research procedures which require expensive equipment.
(1) Total body nitrogen may be measured by in vivo neutron activation with simultaneous counting of the 10·8 MeV γ rays produced from the nitrogen[8]; then $N \times 6·25$ = total body protein.
(2) Total body potassium may be measured by counting in a heavily screened whole body counter the characteristic γ rays from the natural radioisotope ^{40}K which is mixed as 0·012% with the stable ^{39}K isotope throughout our bodies. Potassium is predominantly intracellular and normally proportional to body protein.
(3) Body weight for height partly reflects total protein.
(4) Total protein may also be estimated from the mid-arm muscle circumference (mid-arm circumference $- \pi \times$ triceps skinfold).
(5) 24 Hour urinary creatinine gives a biochemical measure of muscle mass since creatinine is a metabolite from the turnover of muscle creatine. 1 g creatinine/day comes from about 20 kg of muscle but urinary creatinine shows quite large day to day fluctuations even if collection is complete, and it is spuriously increased by eating meat and by exercise.

Visceral protein is sometimes disproportionately reduced in protein deficiency, as seen most strikingly in kwashiorkor. There is fatty liver, intestinal mucosal and pancreatic atrophy, and impaired lymphocyte function. The usual tests are to measure concentrations of plasma albumin or transferrin, proteins synthesised in the liver. Plasma albumin concentrations are also moderately reduced in the metabolic response to severe injury or infection as well as in liver cirrhosis and nephrotic syndrome. Transferrin concentrations are increased in iron deficiency.

Other nutrients do not affect anthropometric measurements directly. Inadequate intake can be suspected from the dietary intake or shown by specific biochemical tests.

Assessment of dietary intake

The sequence of assessing nutrient intake is to
(a) estimate *food intake* as g/day of different foods;
(b) use *food tables* to convert g/day of each individual food to g, mg, or µg/day of various nutrients. These calculations can and always used to be done manually but nutritionists are increasingly using computers;
(c) compare this patient's intake of one or several nutrients likely to be inadequate with the dietary reference values[7] of food energy and nutrients. Note: the reference nutrient intake[7] covers the individual nutrient requirements of the great majority of normal people, which means that an intake somewhat below the recommended daily amount would be adequate for most people (see page 65). The other consideration is whether the day(s) on which food intake was measured were typical.

Food intake measurements

In dietetic work and nutritional surveys four types of method are used. Reliability depends more on attention to detail and the interviewer's knowledge of foods than on the method chosen.
- Dietary history—"What do you eat on a typical day?" This is a good method in the hands of a skilled and patient interviewer. Food models, cups, plates, and spoons are used to estimate portion sizes.
- 24 Hour recall—"Tell me everything you've had to eat and drink in the last 24 hours?" This is less subject to wishful thinking about what the person ought to have eaten. The weakness is that yesterday may have been atypical. 24 Hour recalls can, however, be repeated.

Measuring nutrition

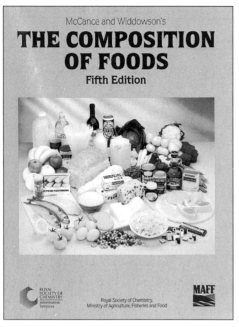

- Food diary or record—"Please write down (and describe) *everything* you eat and drink (and estimate the amount) for the next 3 (4 or 7) days." Amounts are usually recorded in household measures but for more accuracy subjects can be provided with quick reading scales to weigh food before it goes on the plate (and any leftovers).
- Food frequency questionnaire—"Do you eat meat/fish/bread/ milk . . . on average: more than once a day/2 or 3 times a week/once a week/once a month etc?"

Estimating food intake quantitatively is labour intensive (and so expensive). It depends on adequate memory and the honesty and interest of the subject. Some people's food habits are very irregular and most people eat differently on Saturday and Sunday than during the rest of the week and on holiday.

Food tables

The British food tables are among the best in the world thanks to the original work of McCance and Widdowson, their continuation by Paul and Southgate and colleagues, and the support of the Medical Research Council; Ministry of Agriculture, Fisheries, and Food; the Agriculture and Food Research Council; and the Royal Society of Chemistry. The 5th edition of *McCance and Widdowson's The Composition of Foods* was published in 1991,[9] there are five supplements to the 4th edition, and the Royal Society of Chemistry (RSC) will be publishing supplements to the 5th edition (one is already in press) (see box).

In the main volume 1188 foods and drinks arranged in 14 groups are given code numbers (which can be used for computer input – software packages are also available). The total publications, including supplements, cover around 2000 foods. Figures are given (per 100 g edible portion) for most of these foods for the following constituents:

- The proximates or macronutrients – Water, sugars, starch, available carbohydrate, dietary fibre (Southgate method) and non-starch polysaccharides (Englyst method), protein, total nitrogen fat, (alcohol where appropriate), and food energy (in both kcal and kJ).
- Essential inorganic elements – Sodium, potassium, calcium, magnesium, phosphorus, iron, copper, zinc, manganese, iodine, selenium, and chloride.
- Vitamins – A (retinol and carotene), thiamin, riboflavin, niacin (preformed and from tryptophan), B-6, pantothenate, biotin, folate (total), vitamins B-12, C, D, and E.
- Amino acids are given in the first supplement to the 4th edition – For major foods 18 amino acids are given: ile, leu, lys, met, cys, phe, tyr, thr, trp, val, arg, his, ala, asp, glu, gly, pro, and ser.
- Cholesterol and fatty acid fraction totals (saturated, monounsaturated, and polyunsaturated) are given throughout the 5th edition for foods containing fat. Details of 16 or more individual fatty acids can be found in the first supplement to the 4th edition – 14:0, 15:0, 16:0, 17:0, 18:0, 16:1, 18:1, 20:1, 22:1, 18:2, 18:3, 18:4, 20:4, 20:5, 22:5, and 22:6.

Cereals and cereal products *continued*

18 to 32
Composition of food per 100g

No.	Food	Description and main data sources	Edible proportion	Water g	Protein g	Fat g	Carbo-hydrate g	Energy value kcal	kJ
Rice									
18	**Brown rice,** *raw*	5 assorted samples	1.00	13.9	6.7	2.8	81.3	357	1518
19	*boiled*	Water content weighed, other nutrients calculated from raw	1.00	66.0	2.6	1.1	32.1	141	597
20	**Savoury rice,** *raw*	10 samples, 5 varieties, meat and vegetable	1.00	7.0	8.4	10.3	77.4	415	1755
21	*cooked*	Calculation from raw, boiled in water	1.00	68.7	2.9	3.5[a]	26.3	142	599
22	**White rice,** *easy cook, raw*	10 samples, 9 different brands, parboiled	1.00	11.4	7.3	3.6	85.8	383	1630
23	*easy cook, boiled*	Calculation from raw	1.00	68.0	2.6	1.3	30.9	138	587
24	*fried in lard/dripping*	Recipe	1.00	70.3	2.2	3.2	25.0	131	554
Pasta									
25	**Macaroni,** *raw*	10 samples, 7 brands; literature sources	1.00	9.7	12.0	1.8	75.8	348	1483
26	*boiled*	10 samples, 7 brands boiled in water	1.00	78.1	3.0	0.5	18.5	86	365
27	**Noodles,** *egg, raw*	10 samples, 8 brands	1.00	9.1	12.1	8.2	71.7	391	1656
28	*egg, boiled*	10 samples, 8 brands boiled in water	1.00	84.3	2.2	0.5	13.0	62	264
29	**Spaghetti,** *white, raw*	10 samples, 7 brands	1.00	9.8	12.0	1.8	74.1	342	1456
30	*white, boiled*	10 samples, 7 brands boiled in water	1.00	73.8	3.6	0.7	22.2	104	442
31	*wholemeal, raw*	10 samples, 5 brands	1.00	10.5	13.4	2.5	66.2	324	1379
32	*wholemeal, boiled*	Water content weighed, other nutrients calculated from raw	1.00	69.1	4.7	0.9	23.2	113	485

[a] Calculated assuming water only was added; savoury rice cooked with fat contains approximately 8.8g fat per 100g

Cereals and cereal products *continued*

18 to 32
Composition of food per 100g

No.	Food	Total nitrogen g	Fatty acids Satd g	Mono unsatd g	Poly unsatd g	Cholest-erol mg	Starch g	Total sugars g	Dietary fibre Southgate method g	Englyst method g
Rice										
18	**Brown rice,** *raw*	1.10	0.7	0.7	1.0	0	80.0	1.3	3.8	1.9
19	*boiled*	0.43	0.3	0.3	0.4	0	31.6	0.5	1.5	0.8
20	**Savoury rice,** *raw*	1.41	3.2	3.7	1.8	1	73.8	3.6	4.0	N
21	*cooked*	0.48	1.1	1.3	0.6	Tr	25.1	1.2	1.3	1.4
22	**White rice,** *easy cook, raw*	1.23	0.9	0.9	1.3	0	85.8	Tr	2.7	0.4
23	*easy cook, boiled*	0.44	0.3	0.3	0.5	0	30.9	Tr	1.0	0.1
24	*fried in lard/dripping*	0.37	1.4	1.2	0.5	3	23.1	1.9	1.2	0.6
Pasta										
25	**Macaroni,** *raw*	2.11	0.3	0.1	0.8	0	73.6	2.2	5.0	3.1[a]
26	*boiled*	0.52	0.1	Tr	0.2	0	18.2	0.3	1.5	0.9[a]
27	**Noodles,** *egg, raw*	2.12	2.3	3.5	0.9	30	69.8	1.9	5.0	(2.9)
28	*egg, boiled*	0.40	0.1	0.2	0.1	6	12.8	0.2	1.0	(0.6)
29	**Spaghetti,** *white, raw*	2.11	0.2	0.2	0.8	0	70.8	3.3	5.1	2.9
30	*white, boiled*	0.63	0.1	0.1	0.3	0	21.7	0.5	1.8	1.2
31	*wholemeal, raw*	2.30	0.4	0.3	1.1	0	62.5	3.7	11.5	8.4
32	*wholemeal, boiled*	0.81	0.1	0.1	0.4	0	21.9	1.3	4.0	3.5

[a] Wholemeal macaroni contains 8.3g (raw) and 2.8g (boiled) Englyst fibre per 100g

Two pages from *The Composition of Foods*.[9] Each set of foods has four pages of nutrients.

Supplements to *The Composition of Foods*

Amino Acids and Fatty Acids	HMSO, 1980
Immigrant Foods	HMSO, 1985
Cereals and Cereal Products	RSC, 1988
Milk Products and Eggs	RSC, 1989
Vegetables, Herbs and Spices	RSC, 1991
Fruits and Nuts	RSC (in press)

RSC = Royal Society of Chemistry

Thus for most foods there are 75 nutrient substances (41 excluding individual fatty acids and amino acids) in these tables, though there are occasional gaps where analyses have not yet been done. The tables have to be constantly revised as new foods are introduced, the recipes and processing for established foods change, and additional food components are asked for by doctors.

Variability of nutrient content—The British tables give a single value for each nutrient in each food—an estimated average. The American tables,[10] which are published in loose leaf sections as analyses are completed, give an indication of variability to be expected round each average figure. There is no legal guarantee that any food contains what the food tables say it should. For some constituents—for example, fat—the food could easily contain 25% less or 25% more.

Dietary reference values

For nutrient intakes to have any meaning they have to be compared against some number representing physiological requirements for each nutrient. The primary number for this is the estimated upper end of the range of individual requirements. In Britain the name for this was changed in 1991 to *reference nutrient intake* (RNI)[7] from recommended daily amount (RDA). The latter had the same abbreviation as the present American term, recommended dietary allowance[12]; the former has the same abbreviation as recommended nutrient intake, a name we have used in Australia.[13] These different national names imply that this amount of a nutrient is what expert committees recommend people to eat. It is also a reference value.

The RNI/RDA values differ for the two sexes and several age groups and are published in tables.[7 12 13] They are for intakes averaged over several days. Since the RNI/RDA is estimated to meet the requirements of practically all healthy people, most people's requirements are less than this upper or prescriptive reference value. For assessment of people's intakes a lower, diagnostic, reference should be used, such as the *estimated average requirement*.[7] An intake below this does not necessarily mean inadequacy but the lower it is the greater that probability. As elsewhere in medicine, for complete nutritional diagnosis, findings on examination (clinical, anthropometric, and biochemical) must be considered together with the food intake history.

Sick people have requirements not covered by the reference values. For example, with bed rest energy requirements are reduced; with fever they are increased. Losses of several nutrients are increased in different ways by illness, such as protein loss in nephrotic syndrome, potassium loss in diarrhoea, iron loss with bleeding. The allowances apply to oral feeding of conventional foods. For total parenteral nutrition the requirements are different; absorption is 100%, but minor vitamins like pantothenate and biotin and trace elements like molybdenum, manganese, chromium, etc, cannot be taken for granted and have to provided in the infusion solution(s).

Biochemical methods

Biochemical tests are an integral part of modern medical diagnosis. Plasma sodium and potassium concentrations, for example, are essential for diagnosing and treating difficult electrolyte disorders, and plasma or red cell folate and plasma vitamin B-12 should be measured before treating a patient with megaloblastic anaemia.

With most of the other nutrients also biochemical tests have been developed which can be used (*a*) to confirm the diagnosis of a deficiency disease in places where it is uncommonly seen or where the clinical picture is complicated, or (*b*) in community surveys and general practice to find individuals with subclinical nutrient deficiencies.

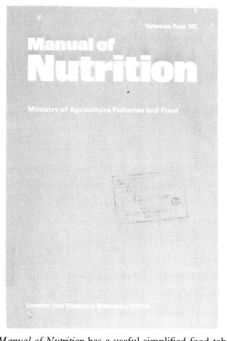

The Manual of Nutrition has a useful simplified food table, which gives calories and 11 nutrients for 150 common foods[11]

British dietary reference values[7]: estimated average requirement for food energy (calories) and reference nutrient intakes (RNIs) for the other nutrients

Nutrient	Men 19–50 years	Infants 4–6 months
Energy, kcal (MJ)	2550 (10·6)	670 (2·8)
Protein (g)	56	13
Vitamin A (RE, μg)	700	350
Thiamin (mg)	1·0	0·2
Riboflavin (mg)	1·3	0·4
Niacin (NE, mg)	17	3
Vitamin B-6 (mg)	1·4	0·2
Folate (total, μg)	200	50
Vitamin B-12 (μg)	1·5	0·3
Vitamin D (μg)	—	8·5
Vitamin E (mg)	7	0·4/g PUF
Calcium (mg)	700	525
Iron (mg)	8·7	4·3
Magnesium (mg)	300	60
Iodine (μg)	140	60
Potassium (mmol)	90	22
Sodium (mmol)	70	12
Zinc (mg)	9·5	4

Some figures are slightly rounded. Figures for women are generally about 75% of those for men, except iron (higher until the menopause) and in pregnancy and lactation. Figures for children are interpolated between infants and adults.
RE = retinol equivalents; NE = niacin equivalents; PUF = polyunsaturated fat.

Measuring nutrition

Principal biochemical methods for diagnosing nutritional deficiencies

Nutrient	Indicating reduced intake	Indicating impaired function (IF) or cell depletion (CD)	Supplementary method
Protein	Urinary nitrogen	Plasma albumin (IF)	Fasting plasma amino acid pattern
Vitamin A	Plasma carotene	Plasma retinol	Relative dose response
Thiamin	Urinary thiamin	Red cell transketolase and TPP effect (IF)	
Riboflavin	Urinary riboflavin	Red cell glutathione reductase and FAD effect (IF)	
Niacin	Urinary N'methyl nicotinamide or 2-pyridone, or both	Red cell NAD/NADP ratio	Fasting plasma tryptophan
Vitamin B-6	Urinary 4-pyridoxic acid	Plasma pyridoxal 5′ phosphate	Urinary xanthurenic acid after tryptophan load
Folate	Plasma folate	Red cell folate (CD)	Urinary FIGLU after histidine load
Vitamin B-12	Plasma holo-transcobalamin II	Plasma vitamin B-12	Schilling test
Vitamin C	Plasma ascorbate	Leucocyte ascorbate (CD)	Urinary ascorbate
Vitamin D	Plasma 25-hydroxy vitamin D	Raised plasma alkaline phosphatase (bone isoenzyme) (IF)	Plasma 1,25 dihydroxy-vitamin D
Vitamin E	Ratio of plasma tocopherol to cholesterol + triglyceride	Red cell haemolysis with H_2O_2 in vitro (IF)	
Vitamin K	Plasma phylloquinone	Plasma prothrombin (IF)	PIVKA II
Sodium	Urinary sodium	Plasma sodium	
Potassium	Urinary potassium	Plasma potassium	Total body potassium by counting ^{40}K
Iron	Plasma iron and transferrin	Plasma ferritin (CD)	Stainable iron in bone marrow
Magnesium	Plasma magnesium	Red cell magnesium (CD)	
Iodine	Urinary (stable) iodine	Plasma thyroxine (IF)	Plasma TSH
Zinc	Plasma zinc	Red cell zinc	

TPP = thiamin pyrophosphate; FAD = flavin adenine dinucleotide; NAD = nicotinamide-adenine-dinucleotide; NADP = NAD phosphate; FIGLU = formiminoglutamic acid; PIVKA II = protein induced by vitamin K absence or antagonist-II; ^{40}K = natural radioactive potassium; TSH = thyroid stimulating hormone.
There are no reliable simple methods for assessing **calcium** status (total body calcium can be measured by in vivo neutron activation analysis).

Tests which can be used for the major nutrients are listed in the table. As with other tests in chemical pathology, there may be false positive and false negative results. For example plasma vitamin B-12 concentrations are increased in acute hepatitis and alkaline phosphatase may not be raised if rickets is accompanied by protein-energy deficiency.

When the intake of a nutrient is inadequate (less than obligatory losses) an individual generally goes through three stages. The first is adaptation to the low intake: urinary excretion of the nutrient or its metabolites typically falls but there is no evidence of abnormal function or of depletion of the cells.

In the second stage there are also biochemical changes indicating either impaired function or cellular depletion, but clinical manifestations of deficiency are absent or non-specific. A good example of a test showing impaired function is red cell transketolase activity. For each blood sample this enzyme is assayed in two test tubes, one with extra thiamin pyrophosphate (TPP), the other without. If the activity is more than 25% higher in the supplemented tube (TPP effect + 25%) this indicates functional thiamin deficiency.

The third stage of depletion is that of clinical deficiency disease.

Most clinical biochemistry laboratories provide only some of the methods in this table as a routine but others could be set up in special circumstances or, alternatively, a laboratory specialising in nutrition research could be asked to help.

1 de Boer JO, van Es AJH, van Raaij JMA, *et al*. Energy requirements and energy expenditure of lean and overweight women, measured by indirect calorimetry. *Am J Clin Nutr* 1987;**46**:13–21.
2 Prentice AM, Black AE, Coward WA, *et al*. High levels of energy expenditure in obese women. *BMJ* 1986;**292**:983.
3 Livingstone MBE, Prentice AM, Coward WA, *et al*. Simultaneous measurement of free-living energy expenditure by the doubly labelled water method and heart-rate monitoring. *Am J Clin Nutr* 1990;52:59–65.
4 Edholm OG, Adam JM, Best TW. Day-to-day weight changes in young men. *Ann Hum Biol* 1974;**1**:3–12.
5 Frisancho AR. New norms of upper limb fat and muscle areas for assessment of nutritional status. *Am J Clin Nutr* 1981;**34**:2540–5.
6 Bishop CW, Bowen PE, Ritchey SJ. Norms for nutritional assessment of American adults by upper arm anthropometry. *Am J Clin Nutr* 1981;**34**:2530–9.
7 Department of Health. *Dietary reference values for food energy and nutrients for the United Kingdom. Report of the panel on dietary reference values of the committee on medical aspects of food policy.* London: HMSO, 1991. (Report on Health and Social Subjects 41.)

8 Allman MA, Allen BJ, Stewart PM, *et al*. Body protein of patients undergoing haemodialysis. *European Journal of Clinical Nutrition* 1990;**44**:123–31.
9 Holland B, Welch AA, Unwin ID, Buss DA, Paul AA, Southgate DAT. *McCance and Widdowson's the composition of foods.* 5th ed. Cambridge: Royal Society of Chemistry, 1991.
10 Human Nutrition Information Service, US Department of Agriculture. *Composition of foods: raw, processed, prepared.* Washington, DC: US Government Printing Office. (21 Agriculture handbooks providing nutrient analyses for over 3600 foods; dairy and egg products 8–1, fast foods 8–21.)
11 Ministry of Agriculture, Fisheries and Food. *Manual of nutrition.* 9th ed. London: HMSO, 1985.
12 Subcommittee on the 10th edition of the RDAs, Food and Nutrition Board, National Research Council. *Recommended dietary allowances.* 10th ed. Washington DC: National Academy Press, 1989.
13 Truswell AS, Dreosti IE, English RM, Palmer N, Rutishauser IHE, eds. *Recommended nutrient intakes: Australian papers.* Mosman, New South Wales: Australian Professional Publications, 1990.

13: THERAPEUTIC DIETS

For the purpose of describing therapeutic alterations to diets a "normal" or average diet provides for a *hypothetical 70 kg man* something like:

Energy 11·3 MJ (2700 kcal)
Protein 13% of energy or 87 g
Fat 35% of energy or about 105 g
Carbohydrates 52% of energy or 350 g

If this hypothetical man has one alcoholic drink a day (60 kcal from alcohol) alcohol will provide 2% of dietary energy and fat and energy come down 1% each.

A "normal" diet provides 75% of these absolute figures for the hypothetical woman (not pregnant or lactating), but the same percentages of energy for the constituents.

The naming of diets

Diets are sometimes described eponymously (Giovanetti diet) or as belonging to a specific disease (renal failure diet). But neither type of name is recommended. Diets named after their (supposed) originator give no clue about their composition and particular diets do not necessarily relate to specific diseases. A "renal failure diet" may also be used for hepatic encephalopathy or rare inborn errors of the ornithine cycle. There have been many "diabetic" and "renal failure" diets.

"Cholesterol lowering diet" is ambiguous (and "low cholesterol diet" is worse). Several diets may lower the plasma concentration of cholesterol—low fat, vegetarian, or increased seed oil (ω6 polyunsaturated fatty acids)—and it is not necessary to lower the *dietary* cholesterol.

The most reliable way of naming diets is by the major change (from an average diet) in its composition.

Sodium

100 mmol Na (2·3 g) is a mild low sodium diet
50 mmol Na (1·2 g) is a moderate low sodium diet
25 mmol Na (0·6 g) is a strict low sodium diet

Protein

50 g/day (0·75 g/kg) is a mild protein restricted diet
30 g/day (0·5 g/kg) is a moderate protein restricted diet
20 g/day (0·33 g/kg) is a severe protein restricted diet

A patient's diet may need to be changed as part of his or her management:
(1) For essential or lifesaving treatment—for example, in coeliac disease, phenylketonuria, galactosaemia, hepatic encephalopathy;
(2) To replete patients who are malnourished because of diseases such as cancer and intestinal diseases;
(3) To produce a negative energy balance in obese people;
(4) As helpful treatment, alternative or complementary to drugs, as in diabetes mellitus, mild hypertension, dyspepsia;
(5) To provide standard conditions for diagnostic tests—for example, for measuring faecal fat, urinary 5-hydroxyindoleacetic acid. Also, an elimination diet is the mainstay in diagnosis of food sensitivity;
(6) To deal with the side effects of some drugs—for example, diets with increased potassium for patients taking long term diuretics or diets with restricted tyramine for patients taking monoamine oxidase inhibiting antidepressants.
(7) Prophylactic diets like those described in chapter 7 on nutrition for adults (dietary goals or guidelines for the general public) often combine mild restriction of energy, fat, and sodium with a moderate increase of dietary fibre.

Therapeutic diets ask patients to make one or more of the following changes: reduce or (virtually) eliminate one or more components, increase one or more food components, change the consistency of the diet, or change the feeding pattern. These are all changes to the patient's usual diet (which, of course, varies somewhat from day to day) or in comparison with a hypothetical "normal" or average diet for the country, culture, age, and sex.

The prescription for a diet should state:
● the nature of the modification(s),
● the degree of each modification,
● the planned duration of these,
● any compensation for essential nutrients compromised by the modifications.

The degree of the modification is as important as the dose in pharmacotherapy. People talk loosely about a "low salt" diet but its sodium intake can range from 25 to 100 mmol/day compared with a normal British sodium intake of over 150 mmol/day.

Likewise with protein, a protein restricted diet may vary from 20 to 50 g/day compared with the standard of about 70 g/day (1 g/kg).

The dietary prescription has to be adjusted for the individual patient:
● for the foods disliked and liked;
● for any sensitivity or intolerance to food;
● for any religious food prohibition (including Ramadan for Moslems, the month when all eating has to be at night);
● for vegetarians;
● to include foods eaten away from home;
● for income, occupation, and level of education;
● for cooking facilities and the patient's domestic situation;

Therapeutic diets

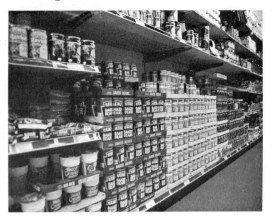

- for the need for variety in foods (some insist on variety; others like the same foods from day to day);
- for the patient's motivation and degree of obsessionality;
- for calorie (energy) expenditure and needs;
- for the duration of the diet. If a diet is necessary for only a week or two then it is not serious if it provides less than the recommended daily amount of (say) calcium or magnesium, but if the diet is continued these elements must be provided, by supplements if necessary;
- for the patient's prognosis. A strict diet may not be justifiable for someone with a short life expectancy;
- when two or more dietary prescriptions are combined. Sometimes these are more or less incompatible—for example a low calorie plus high potassium diet or a high calcium plus lactose free diet (supplements would have to be used for these).

Strategy

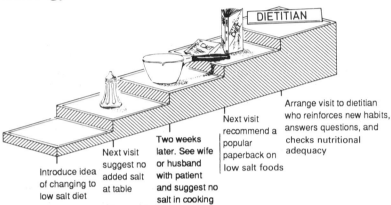

Introduce idea of changing to low salt diet

Next visit suggest no added salt at table

Two weeks later. See wife or husband with patient and suggest no salt in cooking

Next visit recommend a popular paperback on low salt foods

Arrange visit to dietitian who reinforces new habits, answers questions, and checks nutritional adequacy

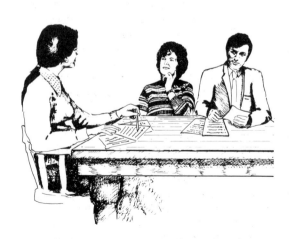

Essential, or lifesaving, diets should be looked after in collaboration with a dietitian.

For some diseases—for example, gout, mild hypertension, dyspepsia, and hyperlipidaemia—drugs or diet are alternative or complementary treatment options. Drugs appear to act more quickly, are easier to administer and more reliable, and take less of the doctor's time, but they may cause more side effects. Diet appears more natural and safer but it will take longer to explain. Sometimes the best choice is a synergistic combination so the dose of drug can be low (hence fewer side effects) and the diet not too irksome.

We know from results with obese people who are on weight reducing diets and from studies in diabetics that most people do not follow the diet prescribed. It is difficult and time consuming to explain what is intended and how it may be done. It is difficult too for a patient to make major changes to his or her food habits. Minor changes are much easier to incorporate and some places in the day's food sequence are easier to change than others. Each family and each individual has different feelings and ideas about foods. Some foods are given up more readily than others.

Outside hospital a therapeutic diet ("I'm on a low salt diet") is a strange association of an occasional talk by the doctor or dietitian with daily action by the patient and his or her family in the supermarket, kitchen, dining room, works canteen, and pub.

Techniques

Essentially the doctor or dietitian has a list of foods rich in the component to be changed and of foods with medium and low amounts of it. The trouble with scientific food tables, such as *McCance and Widdowson's The Composition of Foods*,[1] is that they give the content of nutrients per 100 g whereas what matters is the content per usual serving or portion.

The patient, with his or her spouse, can produce a list of what the family usually eats and how it is cooked. Ideally the next series of steps is for the doctor and these two to work out the most comfortable way for them to incorporate the doctor's prescription into the family's food patterns. This cannot be completed at one session. It requires trial and error, questions and compromises.

There are two fairly easy ways of changing the diet. Firstly, a food that tastes and functions like the original but has a different composition may be substituted. Examples are: polyunsaturated margarine for butter; sunflower (etc) oil for dripping; skimmed or 2% fat milk for whole milk; salt free bread for ordinary bread; wholemeal bread for white bread; high fibre breakfast cereal for a low fibre brand.

Typical serving sizes, approximate weight in grams

Bread (1 slice) 30 g
Crispbread (1 slice)   10 g
Biscuits about 12 g each
Breakfast cereal   30 g
Butter or margarine (for 1 slice bread)   7 g
Oil (1 tablespoonful)   20 g
Cake (portion)   40–50 g
Jam (for 1 slice bread)   15 g
Marmite (for 1 slice bread)   2 g
Milk (for 1 cup tea)   30 g
Milk (6 oz glass)   200 g
Cream (1 tablespoonful)   20 g
Sugar (1 level teaspoon)   5 g
Yoghurt (1 carton)   125–150 g

Cheese (1 portion) 30 g
Egg (1, edible portion) 50 g
Meat (chicken or beef) little or no bone
     90–120 g
Meat (with bone, eg, chop)   160–200 g
Bacon (1 strip, raw)   30–40 g
Liver   100 g
Sausage (one)   50 g (approx)
Fish (fresh and canned)   110–120 g
1 Fish Finger   25 g
Marcaroni and other pasta (for main course)
     100 g (before cooking)
Vegetables (eg, peas, cauliflower)
     60–100 g (before cooking)

Potato (1 medium, raw)   90 g
Lettuce   30g
Parsley (chopped)   3 g
Fruit (1 apple, 1 banana peeled, raw)
     100 g (approx)
1 grape 5 g
Nuts 30 g
Pepper   0·2 g
Wine (glass)   110–125 g
Spirits 25 g
Beer ($\frac{1}{2}$ pint)   285 g
Carbonated soft drink   240–330 g
Coffee powder   2 g

Checking compliance and effectiveness

From an authoritarian viewpoint patients often do not properly comply with the doctor's instructions. This can be checked by asking revealing questions, by calling into the home at meal times, or by biochemical tests.

But for an intelligent patient who thinks that dieting is his or her own responsibility and that of his or her partner, with the doctor as one of their sources of information, what needs to be checked is the effectiveness of what they are doing.

Whatever the viewpoint or words used the same objective tests are available:

● Change of body weight for reduced or increased energy diets,
● Increase of faecal weight for high (wheat) fibre diets,
● 24 Hour urinary sodium and potassium for dietary changes of sodium or potassium,
● 24 Hour urinary nitrogen for high or low protein diets, and also as general check on food intake (on average protein intake is 10–15% of energy intake),
● Plasma fasting triglyceride fatty acid pattern to indicate consumption of polyunsaturated fat,
● Blood urea, urate, glucose, cholesterol, or haemoglobin for respective diets prescribed to moderate these.

Secondly, a simple addition may be made to less important parts of the day's diet. Examples are: a sprinkling of bran on the breakfast cereal to increase fibre; casein powder (such as Casilan) sprinkled on to food three times a day to increase protein; spoonful(s) of fish oil (such as Maxepa) to increase long chain highly polyunsaturated fatty acids.

Diets are more likely to be followed and persisted with by patients who are well motivated, have stable mood, at least normal intelligence, good home support, and lead a well organised life. Indeed, in some obsessional patients there can be the opposite problem of overdoing a diet suggested long ago on thin scientific evidence or for a condition that has since disappeared.

Diets for treating diabetes

History of diets for diabetics 1900–70

1900–25	Fasting (Naunyn, Allen); *5% carbohydrate*, 85% fat (Newburgh 1923)
1922	Insulin discovered (but not generally available for a few years).
1930	*15% carbohydrate* and 70% fat
1940 and 1950	All *carbohydrate low*, eg, 40% and fat 50%. Lawrence's lines in UK.
1970	*Carbohydrate round 40%*; sugar prohibited. Emphasis on oral drugs or insulin rather than diet.

Glycaemic index

Ratio of area under blood glucose curve for two hours after eating food containing 50 g carbohydrate to the corresponding area after ingesting 50 g glucose (measured from the fasting value). For food such as fruit, with a high water content, the amount of carbohydrate tested is 25g.

Since about 1970 the diets used for treating diabetes have undergone further change, as several facts have emerged: (1) Oral hypoglycaemic drugs predispose to heart disease. (2) There is no evidence that eating sugar *causes* diabetes. (3) Asian diabetics on high starch diets have fewer complications (especially atherosclerotic) than their counterparts in Western Europe and North America. (4) Western diabetics are dying of excess atherosclerotic disease, have higher plasma cholesterol values, and have been eating higher fat diets than non-diabetics. (5) Viscous dietary fibres such as that in guar, pectin, and legumes (though carbohydrates) improve diabetic control. (6) Increased dietary carbohydrate improves the response to a glucose tolerance test. Increasing the (complex) carbohydrate of diabetic diets is not usually followed by deteriorating control. (7) Individual foods containing carbohydrate do not give the same glucose and other metabolic responses at a standard intake. When put to the test, amounts containing 50 g carbohydrate of some foods give much higher blood glucose curves than others. They have a higher or lower *glycaemic index*. This means that carbohydrate exchange lists can no longer be relied on. It was always hard to believe that 2 oz of grapes had the same effect in the body as 7 oz of whole milk. The main cause of a low glycaemic index is that the starch in the food is digested slowly by pancreatic amylase. (8) Diabetics also have an increased chance of developing hypertension. The sodium content of their diets has been largely ignored.

Therapeutic diets

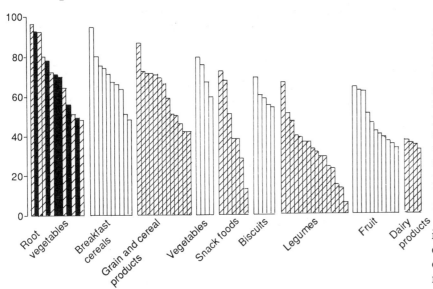

Reported glycaemic indices for single foods arranged in groups, based on reports from six research groups. The solid bars represent one food—potatoes.

The British Diabetic Association recommends that diabetic diets should contain 55% of calories as carbohydrate, as much as possible unrefined and starchy. Fat should be about 35% of calories (a little less than the average consumption in Britain) with saturated fat most restricted. The association sees little place for sorbitol and fructose, which contain as much chemical energy as other carbohydrates. Non-caloric sweeteners like saccharin are useful. Diabetics should not be prescribed a diet that contains more sodium than that consumed by non-diabetics. Current recommendations in the USA are similar.

In practice about 90% of diabetics have non-insulin dependent diabetes, usually maturity onset, and they are usually overweight. The overwhelming objective in their dietary management is to reduce weight by combining a low energy diet with increased exercise.

In insulin dependent diabetics food should be distributed in the day to match the times of greatest insulin activity. Distribution and amounts should be kept as constant as possible from day to day. The emphasis should be on foods low in fat with a low glycaemic index.

Aim for non-insulin dependent diabetics

Reduce weight by combining a low energy intake from a balanced diet low in fat, alcohol, and sugar with increased exercise

---

In a three month/three month crossover trial a diet of palatable low glycaemic index (GI) foods was compared with a usual Western diet (processed cereals, potatoes, etc). Glycosylated haemoglobin, diurnal plasma glucose, and urinary glucose were all lower on the low GI diet.[2]

Foods that have been shown to have low glycaemic indices (15 to 50) compared with glucose (glycaemic index = 100)

Soya beans	Pearl barley	Cherries
Lentils	Pastas (white)	Plums
Dried peas	Pastas (wholemeal)	Apples
Canned baked beans	Porridge oats	Apple juice
Frozen peas	All Bran	Grapefruit
Other dried legumes	Pumpernickel bread	Oranges
		Orange juice
Milk (full cream or skimmed) and yoghurt		Peaches

High fat foods may also give a low glycaemic index, because of delayed gastric emptying, but are not in this list and not recommended

---

Diets for renal failure

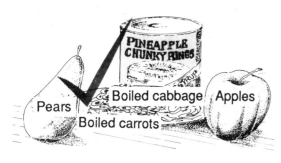

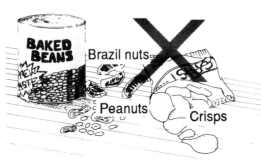

A strict therapeutic diet is needed for patients with renal failure during the few days between diagnosis and dialysis and for the minority for whom dialysis will not be used. The diet should be low in protein (40 g/day) or very low in high biological value protein (25 g/day) with low potassium and a controlled sodium and water intake.

Most patients with chronic renal failure in Western countries are, however, nowadays treated with regular dialysis while awaiting a transplant. For them the outpatient diet is not very different from a normal one. Protein should be about 1·2 g/kg body weight, a little more than the recommended daily intake for healthy people. Rather more protein is lost, and so needed, on continuous ambulatory peritoneal dialysis than on haemodialysis. Potassium is carefully monitored but usually needs to be only a little restricted, sometimes not at all. It is controlled by adjusting the concentration in the dialysing fluid; 50 mmol/day is an average amount for the diet. This is achieved by eating fruits which have a low potassium content (apples, pears, and canned fruits) and boiled leafy vegetables and avoiding higher potassium vegetables (legumes), nuts, dried fruits, chocolate, and potato chips and crisps.

Patients can usually take an ordinary amount of sodium (about 110 mmol/day) or need only mild restriction. Fluid intake is restricted to about 1000 ml/day. Supplements of water soluble vitamins should not be given above nutrient requirement dosage.[3] Fat soluble vitamin supplements are not required; they tend to accumulate.

Other conditions

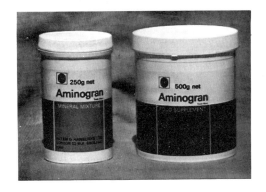

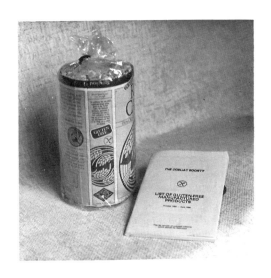

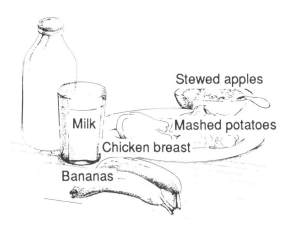

Milk
Stewed apples
Mashed potatoes
Chicken breast
Bananas

Phenylketonuria is one of the better known examples of an inborn error of amino acid metabolism. It leads to mental retardation and other abnormalities if patients are not started on a low phenylalanine diet in the first few weeks of life. Diagnosis is by routine screening of blood phenylalanine after adequate intakes of milk, on about the seventh day of life. Bottle feeding is essential in infancy and a special low phenylalanine formula has to be used, such as Lofenalac or Minafen. When the child is weaned the diet has to be very different from that of other children: a combination of low protein foods and a phenylalanine free mixture of other essential amino acids—for example, Aminogran— with sugars and fats. The relative amounts of the first two are adjusted to maintain plasma phenylalanine neither too high (toxicity) nor too low (inadequate growth). The diet has to be strictly maintained and monitored until the child is about 8 years old, after which it can usually be relaxed. But it is required again in women during pregnancy.

Patients with *gluten sensitive enteropathy*, coeliac disease, and dermatitis herpetiformis have to modify their diets to eliminate all wheat gluten, rye and barley gluten, and possibly oats. Fresh milk, fresh meat, fish and eggs, fresh vegetables and fruit, rice and maize, tea, coffee, sugar, wine, and spirits are all safe but many processed foods have wheat flour or gluten added. With many of these foods some brands contain gluten, others do not. The only thing to do is to check ingredients on the label or check brands against an up to date copy of the Coeliac Society's list of gluten free manufactured products (PO Box 181, London NW2 2QY). Gluten free breads and pasta and other products, even communion wafers, are available, some on prescription. Unlike many other diets, even a small lapse and inclusion of the harmful component can lead to prompt return of symptoms.

Diets for dyspepsia present a contrast to the two preceding essential diets. Classic diets for peptic ulcer have not been found to accelerate healing in controlled barium meal studies; modern drug treatment, especially with H_2 receptor antagonists, insoluble alkalis, or bismuth compounds, is usually effective. Diet is therefore less emphasised than before for gastroduodenal diseases. Nevertheless, some foods are known to cause gastric irritation or stimulate acid secretion, including chili powder, coffee, tea, peppers, alcohol, and cola beverages. Other foods commonly cause heartburn by lowering the tone of the lower oesophageal sphincter: peppermint, garlic, onion, fatty meals. Frequent, small volume feeds are beneficial in both peptic ulcer and oesophageal reflux. Traditional bland foods such as milk, chicken, mashed potatoes, bananas, apples, and ice cream usually relieve symptoms in patients with dyspepsia, though individuals vary.

Glucose tolerance tests
Faecal fat test
Urinary screening for hypercalciuria
5-hydroxyindoleacetic acid (5-HIAA)
4-hydroxy-3-methoxy-mandelic acid (VMA)
Creatinine

Diets for diagnostic tests—For several days before a *glucose tolerance test* patients should be standardised on enough carbohydrate—that is, about 300 g or at least 50% of calories, the amount of carbohydrate in ordinary Western diets. Before a *faecal fat* test for malabsorption patients should be on a known, controlled, and adequate fat intake, 70 to 100 g/day. Before *urinary screening for hypercalciuria* patients should be on a high normal calcium intake of about 1000 mg/day. Before urine is collected for 5-*hydroxyindoleacetic acid* (5-HIAA) measurement dietary sources of it or of serotonin should be excluded: bananas, plantains, tomatoes, plums, avocadoes, pineapples, passion fruit, and walnuts. For urinary *4-hydroxy-3-methoxy-mandelic acid* (VMA) specific laboratory methods are now used, and dietary preparation should be unnecessary. Even urinary *creatinine* is affected (increased) by meat consumption.

Therapeutic diets

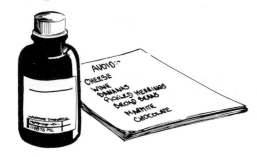

1 Holland B, Welch AA, Unwin ID, Buss DA, Paul AA, Southgate DAT. *McCance and Widdowson's the composition of foods*. 5th ed. Cambridge: Royal Society of Chemistry, 1991.
2 Brand JC, Colagiuri S, Crossman S, Allen A, Roberts DCK, Truswell AS. Low-glycemic index foods improve long-term glycemic control in NIDDM. *Diabetes Care* 1991; **14**: 95–101.
3 Allman MA, Truswell AS, Stewart PM, Yan DF, Tiller DJ, *et al*. Vitamin supplementation of patients receiving haemodialysis. *Med J Aust* 1989;**150**:130–3.

Further reading

Jenkins DJA, Wolever TMS, Jenkins AL. Starchy foods and glycemic index. *Daibetes Care* 1988;**11**:149–59.
Thomas B, ed. *Manual of dietetic practice*. (British Dietetic Association). Oxford: Blackwell Scientific, 1988.
Crawley H. *Food portion sizes*. London: HMSO (Ministry of Agriculture, Fisheries, and Food), 1988.

Diet for patients taking monoamine oxidase inhibitors—The diet for depressed patients taking these antidepressants is the most striking example of dietary adjustment to prevent side effects from drugs. Monoamine oxidase inhibitors interfere with the normal breakdown of tyramine, dopamine, and other amines that occur naturally in foods in which flavour is enhanced by protein breakdown. Dangerous increases of blood pressure may follow ingestion of cheddar cheese, but other foods contain these amines and should be excluded too: wines, bananas, aged game, pickled herrings, broad beans, and yeast and meat extracts. The drugs which require this dietary modification include tranylcypromine, phenelzine, and isocarboxazid.

In practice the most commonly needed diet is one with reduced energy and the second most needed is a regimen with reduced alcohol intake. Both are prescribed much more often than they are successfully followed. This discrepancy remains a challenge for medical practice and research.

Elsewhere in this book are described diets low in energy (calories) (chapter 11); with altered potassium (chapter 2); low in sodium (chapter 2); low in oxalate (chapter 3); low in saturated fat, with increased polyunsaturated fat (chapter 1); and elimination diets (chapter 16).

14: ENTERAL AND PARENTERAL NUTRITION

MILES H IRVING

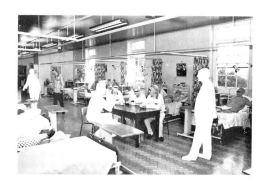

Patients in hospital have a high risk of nutritional disorders, a risk that rises with increasing length of stay. Some patients are admitted with an illness that has caused the problem. Others develop nutritional complications whilst undergoing treatment. Bistrian and Blackburn considered that 44% of general medical[1] and 50% of general surgical patients[2] in the wards of an American municipal hospital had some features of protein-energy malnutrition. Hill found that 26% of patients in the surgical wards of the Leeds General Infirmary were hypoalbuminaemic.[3] Although minor degrees of protein-energy malnutrition do not appear to affect the outcome of surgical operation major nutritional disorders undoubtedly jeopardise recovery.

As many as half the patients on a general surgical ward may show some manifestation of protein malnutrition. The incidence of protein-energy malnutrition rises in patients who stay in hospital for over two weeks.[4]

Types of malnutrition in hospital patients

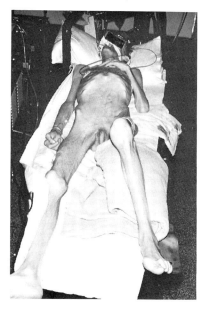

Surgical patients with septic complications tend to have a kwashiorkor-like malnutrition characterised by a low serum albumin concentration, muscle wasting, and water retention. On the other hand, medical patients tend towards marasmus. Most patients who develop a nutritional problem after operation have a mixed picture resulting from starvation, increased catabolism, and reduced anabolism. Malnutrition in surgical patients is accompanied by an increased risk of postoperative complications.

Protein-energy malnutrition resulting from a combination of sepsis and starvation induced by an intestinal fistula.

Detecting malnutrition

Some criteria of malnutrition in inpatients

10% Recent unintentional weight loss
Body weight <80% of ideal for height
Serum albumin less than 30 g/l
Total lymphocyte count of less than $1.2 \times 10^6/1$

Many methods of detecting protein-energy malnutrition have been advanced, varying from the sophisticated to the simple. Those requiring complex equipment, such as neutron activation analysis for measuring total body nitrogen, are research tools. Valuable information can be obtained from simpler measurements such as change in body weight, arm muscle circumference, and serum albumin concentration. These can, however, be difficult to interpret in the short term because of complicating factors such as water retention. Once malnutrition is detected, treatment should be started to reverse it. Nutritional treatment will not be effective in the presence of active sepsis. The priority in such cases is to eliminate the septic focus.

Enteral and parenteral nutrition

Treating malnutrition

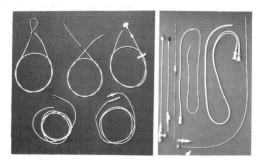

Nutrients can be administered direct into the gastrointestinal tract—that is, enteral nutrition—or into the blood stream—that is, parenteral nutrition. Parenteral nutrition is indicated only when enteral feeding is not feasible. Only a few patients are unsuitable for enteral nutrition.

Left: fine bore nasogastric feeding tubes. Right: silastic catheters used for semipermanent implantation into superior vena cava via subclavian vein.

Enteral nutrition

Indications for enteral nutrition

Unconsciousness
Neurological dysphagia
Oesophageal obstruction
Inflammatory bowel disease
Short bowel syndrome
Post-traumatic weakness
Postoperative weakness
Post irradiation weakness
Head and neck surgery
Chemotherapy
Burns
Old age

Enteral nutrition using chemically defined liquid regimens should be prescribed when patients cannot eat sufficient normal food. Enteral nutrition can be total or supplemental. Supplemental feeding is used when a patient needs an easily taken nutrient preparation to supplement an inadequate intake of normal food. Total enteral nutrition is primarily indicated in patients who cannot eat or drink because of unconsciousness, partial obstruction or disease of the intestinal tract, or inability to swallow because of neurological disorders. Some patients need enteral nutrition with a liquid diet because they cannot swallow solids or because of high losses from fistulas or stomas.

Administration of total enteral nutrition

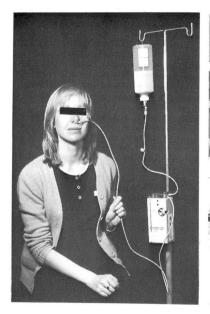
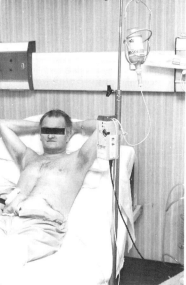

In some patients who cannot eat because of dysphagia the normal diet may be liquidised and swallowed in the usual way. Alternatively a commercially prepared liquid food may be used. Patients who cannot swallow or those with continually high losses from stomas or fistulas will need tube feeding.

Modern feeding tubes are of fine bore and made of polyurethane or silastic. They are easily tolerated by the patient and can remain in position for long periods without damaging the oesophagus. Their fine bore precludes their use for the administration of liquidised food; only the commercially available chemically defined preparations can be easily administered through them. In patients with total oesophageal obstruction or upper intestinal fistulas the diet can be infused directly into the jejunum through a fine tube jejunostomy.

Left: fine bore nasogastric feeding tube in position with direct administration from container. Right: patient with gastric outlet obstruction and duodenal fistula being fed through a fine bore jejunostomy tube.

Choice of enteral nutrient

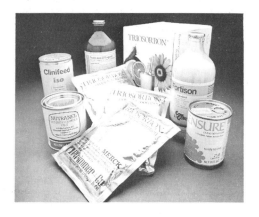

There is a wide range of enteral preparations, the principal differences between them being in the way the protein and energy are presented. Liquid whole protein regimens are cheaper and more palatable than those based on oligopeptides and amino acids.

The oligopeptide and amino acid preparations are alleged to be better absorbed, especially in patients with shortened or diseased bowel. But there is no good evidence that this is so, and the preparation of choice for routine use is a whole protein regimen. The energy content of the diet is offered as glucose, oligosaccharides, maltodextrin, corn syrup, medium chain triglycerides, sunflower oil, etc. Other essential nutrients, such as electrolytes, minerals, trace elements, and vitamins, are added in varying quantities, depending on the preparation. Several diets do not contain lactose and can be used in patients with lactose intolerance. Variations of the basic formula allow for increased energy and nitrogen provision or reduced sodium content.

Composition of an ideal enteral diet—
An average patient will need 8·4–12·6 MJ (2000–3000 kcal) and 10–15 g nitrogen, corresponding to 60–90 g protein in 2–3 litres of fluid. The proportion of energy provided by fat should be about 30–40%. The mixture should contain essential minerals, trace elements, and vitamins.

Complications of enteral feeding

Simply because an enteral regimen is being administered into the gastrointestinal tract it cannot be assumed that the treatment is relatively free of complications. Patients receiving this treatment are at risk from aspiration, vomiting, diarrhoea, and disturbances of metabolism and water balance. Additionally, careless handling of the regimen can result in it becoming infected.

Components of typical whole protein polymeric liquid enteral diet

Water	Coconut oil
Sodium caseinate	Lecithin
Calcium caseinate	Minerals
Maltodextrin	Trace elements
Corn oil	Vitamins
Palm oil	

500 ml of this diet provides 20 g protein (3·15 g nitrogen) and 2·1 MJ (500 kcal)

Complications of enteral feeding

Gastric retention	Hyperosmolar coma
Aspiration	Hyperglycaemia
Nausea and vomiting	Tube misplacement
Diarrhoea	Oesophageal erosions
Dehydration	Infection

Ambulatory home enteral nutrition

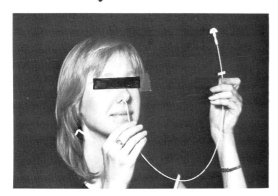

In some patients the need for nutrients is so high that continuous administration is necessary. Others can only cope with their requirements by prolonged nutrition. Such patients can be taught to insert feeding tubes themselves and assemble their infusion for overnight administration or alternatively feed themselves by continuous infusion using a portable pump. This allows them to go home from hospital and resume a more normal life, including going to work.

Patient inserting fine bore feeding tube into stomach for continuous overnight intragastric infusion

Parenteral nutrition

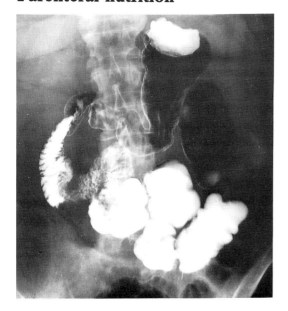

Intravenous administration of nutrients is indicated when patients cannot be fed by mouth, by nasogastric intubation, or by jejunostomy. Such patients can be said to be in a state of "intestinal failure". This condition may be defined as "the reduction of functioning gut mass below the amount necessary for adequate digestion and absorption of nutrients."[5] [6] Intestinal failure may be acute and reversible, for example, until a fistula closes or a segment of short bowel adapts. Alternatively it may be chronic, as in patients with short bowel syndrome, from whom virtually all ileum and jejunum have been removed.

Barium meal in patient with short bowel syndrome. Duodenocolic anastomosis after total excision of small bowel.

Enteral and parenteral nutrition

Technique of parenteral nutrition

Access to the circulation for intravenous feeding can be by a peripheral vein. But even when isotonic solutions are used, the veins tend to thrombose, making this method one for only short term use. For long term intravenous feeding the catheter is best introduced into a major vein such as the subclavian, the tip being advanced until it lies in the superior vena cava. The remainder of the catheter is tunnelled in the subcutaneous tissues to emerge on the anterior chest wall.

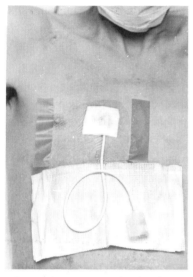 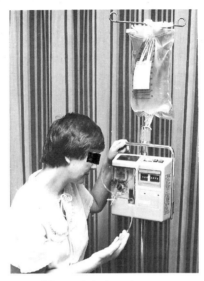

With careful attention to asepsis and the use of antiseptic dressings infections can be prevented and the catheters can remain in situ indefinitely. Although in the early stages parenteral nutrition is given throughout the day, once a patient's condition stabilises the feed may be given just during the night. During the day the catheter can be filled with heparin, thereby allowing the patient to move around normally.

Nutrients are administered to the patient from a 3 litre bag, which is filled in the pharmacy under sterile conditions. A regular rate of infusion is ensured by using a constant volume infusion pump, which incorporates alarms to warn of air in the infusion system and changes in the flow rate.

Left: silastic catheter running in subcutaneous tunnel from subclavian vein to emerge on chest wall. Right: constant volume infusion pump for continuous administration of nutrient. Three litre bag contains 24 h requirements of water, electrolytes, amino acids, energy (calories), trace elements, and vitamins.

Nutrients used in parenteral feeding

The regimen used is broadly tailored to an individual's requirements. A stable patient with intestinal failure usually requires about 10·5 MJ (2500 kcal) of energy and 12 g of nitrogen as crystalline amino acids in 2500 ml of fluid. Energy is provided using glucose and lipid emulsion. In the United Kingdom the latter is a soya bean oil emulsion which seems to have the same properties as chylomicrons. In patients in hospital lipid usually provides about 30% of the calories infused.

Amino acid provision includes all the essential amino acids, and a wide range of non-essential ones. The ratio of amino acids one to another—the aminogram—usually approximates that of a high quality protein such as egg albumin.

Mixed into the bag with the above are the normal daily requirement of electrolytes, trace elements, and vitamins. For patients in an unstable condition with increased catabolism and sepsis, the regimen has to be modified to take into account the increased requirements for vitamin B complex, trace elements, and electrolytes. Treatment with parenteral nutrition continues until the underlying condition has resolved and enteral nutrition can be reintroduced.

Intravenous amino acid solutions, glucose, fat, vitamin, and trace metal supplements used in total parenteral nutrition.

Complications of parenteral nutrition

The principal complication of parenteral nutrition is infection of the intravenous feeding catheter, which can produce septicaemia. If this happens the catheter must be removed.

Thrombosis of the vessel into which the infusion is being delivered can occur. Extravasation of the infused fluid due to misplacement of the catheter tip is preventable by screening at the time of placing the catheter.

Metabolic problems such as hyperglycaemia can arise from infusion of the glucose load, although this usually settles as the patient's body adapts to this form of treatment. In the long term trace element deficiencies can create problems but these are preventable by careful monitoring.

Ambulatory home parenteral nutrition

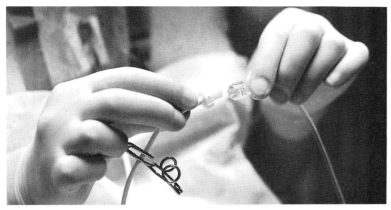

Patient on home parenteral nutrition connecting herself to infusion.

In patients in whom restoration of enteral nutrition is likely to be delayed or in those committed to lifelong support by parenteral feeding the advantages of home parenteral nutrition should be considered. Patients can be taught the techniques of catheter care and intravenous infusion. This enables them to leave hospital and return to the community. Most of these patients, by feeding themselves overnight, can live an active social life and return to work.

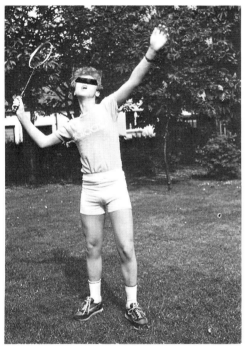

A good quality of life can be achieved by home parenteral nutrition. This fit 16 year old is in his second year on home parenteral nutrition after duodenocolic anastomosis occasioned by total loss of the small bowel resulting from volvulus.

In the United Kingdom over the past 13 years 350 patients have been trained in this technique, most in centres specialising in its use. A few are now completing their 10th year of treatment. Principal centres in the United Kingdom providing facilites for home parenteral nutrition are, in order of experience, Hope Hospital, Salford; St Mark's Hospital, London; King's Cross Hospital, Dundee; Royal Victoria Infirmary and the Freeman Hospital, Newcastle upon Tyne; Northern General Hospital, Sheffield.

1 Bistrian BR, Blackburn GL, Vitale J, Cochran D, Nayla J. Prevalence of malnutrition in general medical patients. *JAMA* 1976;**235**:1567–70.
2 Bistrian BR, Blackburn GL, Hallowell E, Heddle R. Protein status of general surgery patients. *JAMA* 1974;**230**:858–60.
3 Hill GL, Pickford I, Young GA, *et al*. Malnutrition in surgical patients: an unrecognised problem. *Lancet* 1981;i:689–92.
4 Weinsier RL, Butterworth CE. *Handbook of clinical nutrition*, ch 1. St Louis: CV Mosby, 1981:6
5 Fleming CR, Remington M. Nutrition and the surgical patient. In: Hill GL, ed. *Clinical surgery interntional*. London: Churchill Livingstone, 1981:219–35.
6 Silk DBA. *Nutritional support in hospital practice*. Oxford: Blackwell, 1983.

Further reading
Dretsky AS. Parenteral nutrition – is it helpful? *N Engl J Med* 1991;**325**:573–5.

15: FOOD POISONING

NORMAN D NOAH

> An acute illness, which usually includes one or more gastrointestinal symptoms, caused by the recent consumption of food or drink
>
> Typhoid, paratyphoid, and hepatitis A are not usually considered to be food poisoning

Organisms cause food poisoning by direct invasion of the wall of the intenstine—for example, salmonella—or by production of an enterotoxin—for example, *Clostridium perfringens, Staphylococcus aureus.* The chief sources of data on food poisoning in England and Wales are statutory notifications, and reports from laboratories and departments of environmental health to the Communicable Disease Surveillance Centre.

Food poisoning is a statutorily notifiable disease but is considerably undernotified, with 4500 to more than 39 000 (in 1989) cases formally notified to the Office of Population Censuses and Surveys each year.

Food poisoning generally is commoner in hot weather, although cases are reported throughout the year.

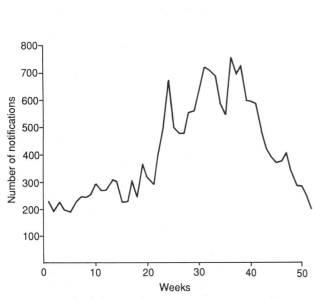

Food poisoning: weekly notifications England and Wales, 1987 (week 30 is late in July)

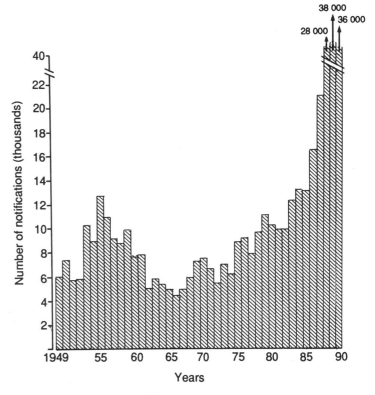

Food poisoning: annual notifications England and Wales, 1949–89

Causes of food poisoning

Microbiological	Chemical including		
	Vegetable	*Fish/shellfish*	*Others include*
Bacterial	Red beans	Scombrotoxin	Heavy metals
Viral	Mushroom/	Ciguatoxin	Monosodium
Protozoal	other fungal	(dinoflagellates)	glutamate
	Solanine	?Domoic acid	Orthotricresyl
		Other toxins	phosphate
			Pesticides

Although this chapter deals mainly with microbiological food poisoning, other causes of food poisoning and acute non-foodborne infectious gastroenteritis will be considered where relevant in the differential diagnosis.

Outbreaks—Within the family, outbreaks of salmonella food poisoning are reported far more often than any other type. Outside the family salmonellas are still the most common, but *C perfringens* outbreaks also account for a high proportion. *Staph aureus* and *Bacillus* spp are less common and *Vibrio parahaemolyticus* rare. Food poisoning from scombrotoxin and red kidney beans has only been recognised in recent years. Red bean food poisoning is now rarely reported.

Laboratory reported outbreaks 1975–86*

	General	Family
Salmonellas	1601	3742
C perfringens	722	40
S aureus	110	48
Bacillus cereus/sp	143	18
V parahaemolyticus	5	1

Other incidents†	
Red beans	17
Scombrotoxin	13
Unknown/viral	216

* England and Wales. † Since 1979 only. All numbers are provisional

Differential diagnosis

Short incubation period

Staph aureus	2–6 h
B cereus (emetic type)	1–5 h
B licheniformis	2–14 h
B subtilis	10 min–14 h
Red beans	1–3 h
Solanine	1–3 h
Heavy metals eg Zn, Cu, Cd, As	5 min–2 h
Scombrotoxin	10–60 min
Ciguatoxin (dinoflagellates)	5 min–4 h
Mushrooms	Few minutes to
Amanita muscaria (fly agaric),	6 h (muscarinic),
	6–24 h (amanitinic)
A pantherina (panther cap, false blusher)	

Medium incubation period

Salmonellas	12–36 h (range 6–48 h)
C perfringens	8–24 h
C botulinum	12–36 h (usually but range from 6–8 days)
V parahaemolyticus	12–24 h (2–48 h)
B cereus (diarrhoeal type)	8–16 h
Mushrooms	6–24 h
A phalloides (death cap); A verna (spring amanita, fool's mushroom); A virosa (destroying angel)	

Long incubation period

Occasionally foodborne

Campylobacters	2–5 days
Small round structured viruses	36–72 h

Rarely food or waterborne

E coli	12–72 h
enteroinvasive (EIEC)	
enteropathogenic (EPEC)	
enterotoxigenic (ETEC)	
enterohaemorrhagic (EHEC)	
Y enterocolitica	2–10 days
Cryptosporidium	4–12 days
G lamblia	1–4 weeks
E histolytica	1–4 weeks
Rotaviruses	1–7 days
Listeria	48 h–?Several weeks

Outbreaks of unknown cause account for a significant proportion of all general outbreaks, but recently some of these have been shown to be viral in origin.

Location of outbreaks—Salmonella food poisoning is fairly ubiquitous; outbreaks in hospitals may be particularly difficult to manage as point source (caused by one meal) outbreaks often lead to transmission from person to person among patients and staff. In 1979–86 the Communicable Disease Surveillance Centre received reports of 168 outbreaks in hospitals; psychiatric and geriatric hospitals were apparently particularly vulnerable. Clostridial food poisoning outbreaks tend to be reported mainly in association with mass catering: restaurants and receptions, hospitals, institutions, canteens. *B cereus* is most often reported in outbreaks associated with Chinese restaurants (fried rice).

The differential diagnosis may be conveniently considered by the length of the incubation period, which may be short, medium, or long.

Food poisoning of *short incubation* tends to be toxic in origin. The enterotoxin of *Staph aureus* and the emetic toxin of *B cereus* are not as a rule destroyed by boiling, though prolonged boiling may denature staphylococcal enterotoxin. Red beans are toxic only when eaten raw, and the toxin is thought to be a haemagglutinin similar to ricin. Scombrotoxin is a histamine like substance released in the flesh of certain fish such as mackerel, herring, and tuna by the effect of enzymes and bacteria. Ciguatoxin may be found in the flesh of tropical fish; the toxin is produced by a dinoflagellate on which fish may feed. Other types of poisoning from fish have been described. The toxin of the dinoflagellate plankton *Gonyaulax tamarensis* in mussels may cause paralytic shellfish poisoning at certain times ("red tide"). Solanine is found in green potatoes and is not denatured by cooking. It may be leached out by boiling, as it is water soluble, but not by baking. Food poisoning due to heavy metals characteristically brings on acute vomiting in less than half an hour (and should be considered particularly when this occurs). Cooking food (especially fruit) or serving acidic or alcoholic drinks in, for example, a galvanised pan may lead to metal poisoning. Pesticides applied inappropriately (eg aldicarbs to watermelons and cucumbers) may cause food poisoning.

Medium incubation period—The salmonellas and vibrios cause gastroenteritis by their invasive properties, the others by toxin. The salmonellas may invade the body and cause bacteraemia, meningitis, osteomyelitis, multiple abscesses, and other sepsis. *C perfringens* types A, C, and D may all produce an enterotoxin which is heat labile, though only type A is implicated in food poisoning in the UK. *C perfringens* and possibly *B cereus* (diarrhoeal type) produce their toxins in the intestine rather than in the food, while *B cereus* (emetic type) and *Staph aureus* produce their toxins in food. *C botulinum* produces its toxins in food, but may also produce some toxin in the intestine and, in infant botulism, probably solely in the intestine. *C botulinum* intoxication causes vomiting, sometimes abdominal pain, but not diarrhoea, before causing its characteristic, and often fatal, acute neurological syndrome. Life can be saved with prolonged ventilatory support and intensive care. Fresh food rarely conveys botulism: some cooking or preserving is required for the organism to grow, which it does under anaerobic conditions. Nevertheless, the toxin is heat labile, and also sensitive to pH and chemicals; toxin production is less likely at pH > 4·5 or in the presence of nitrite.

Long incubation period—All these organisms may cause gastroenteritis, but this is not often foodborne. The campylobacters are now the commonest identified group of organisms causing acute gastroenteritis reported to the Communicable Disease Surveillance Centre, with more than 27 000 infections recorded by the unit in 1987. Most cases are apparently sporadic and their source unknown. When outbreaks do occur they are usually traced to unpasteurised milk or contaminated water and only rarely to poultry, even though campylobacters can often be grown from poultry carcasses. A dysentery like syndrome is characteristic of campylobacter enteritis.

Food poisoning

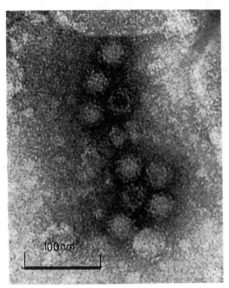

Small round structured viruses (Norwalk agent)

Small round structured viruses are sometimes referred to as Norwalk agent. A very small dose is required for symptoms to occur, and a symptomatic food handler is the usual source of contamination of food. Any food vehicle may transmit the infection in this way. Molluscan shellfish may also be infected, usually by water contaminated with sewage. Constitutional symptoms such as malaise and fever are common and diarrhoea may not be especially prominent. Small round structured viruses share certain properties with hepatitis A virus—namely, a small dose produces symptoms, they are resistant to gastric acid, humans act as carriers but only transiently, and shellfish is a common vehicle.

Escherichia coli is a common cause of gastroenteritis (travellers' diarrhoea, infantile diarrhoea) but outbreaks have only occasionally been attributed to foods: these include cheese and beefburgers (EHEC). *Giardia lamblia* is also a common cause of gastroenteritis but is rarely foodborne, although waterborne outbreaks have occurred. In Britain amoebic dysentery is rarely foodborne or waterborne.

Cryptosporidium is a coccidial protozoan parasite and infection has only rarely been shown to be foodborne (raw tripe). *Yersinia enterocolitica* enteritis tends to affect children and babies, but foodborne disease does occur (milk). Rotavirus infection is very rarely foodborne. *Listeria monocytogenes* may contaminate unpasteurised milk and cheese (especially soft cheese), raw vegetables, raw meat, and seafoods. Pregnant women, fetuses, neonates, and immunosuppressed or elderly patients are especially at risk. *Shigella* spp and parvoviruses have also been incriminated in outbreaks of food poisoning.

Diagnosis

Specimens to send

Specimen:	Test for
Vomit	— *Staph aureus*
	— *B cereus*
	— *B subtilis*
	— heavy metals
Stools	— food poisoning bacteria
	— viruses (electron microscopy only)
	— toxins (*C perfringens*)
	— giardia/amoebae (light microscopy)
	— cryptosporidium (light microscopy)
Foods	— food poisoning bacteria
	— toxins (*Staph aureus*, *C botulinum*, and *B cereus*)
Serum	— toxin (*C botulinum*)
	— viruses (see below)
	— *Y enterocolitica*
Blood/CSF	— *L monocytogenes*

CSF = cerebrospinal fluid

The diagnosis may be suspected from the clinical features, incubation period (if the food vehicle and time of consumption are known), and type of food.

The diagnosis may be made by sending appropriate specimens to a laboratory. These may include foods. Send faecal specimens during the acute phase or as soon as possible afterwards (especially important for viruses). Clostridial enterotoxin is most likely to be detected in specimens of faeces sent within two days of onset.

Bacterial tests on stools and foods

Toxin detection:
 Staph aureus (food only)
 B cereus (diarrhoea enterotoxin —food only)
 C perfringens (faeces only)
 C botulinum (foods, faeces, also serum)

Counts:

 B cereus
 B licheniformis   organisms > 10⁵
 B subtilis   or 10⁶/g in food
 C perfringens   or faeces
 Staph aureus (foods)

Culture:
 Salmonellas (food or faeces)
 All other bacteria (food or faeces)

Typing:
 Salmonellas (serotyping; some types only, eg *Salm typhimurium* for phage typing; patterns of resistance to antibiotics)
 C perfringens (serotyping)
 B cereus (serotyping)
 Staphylococci (enterotoxin tests types A–E; phage typing)
 Campylobacters (serotyping)

Bacteriological tests on stools and foods—The usual method of detecting bacteria is by culture. With common organisms, however, further typing may be necessary—for example with *Salm typhimurium* tests for phage typing, antibiotic resistance patterns, or ability to transfer resistance may be performed.

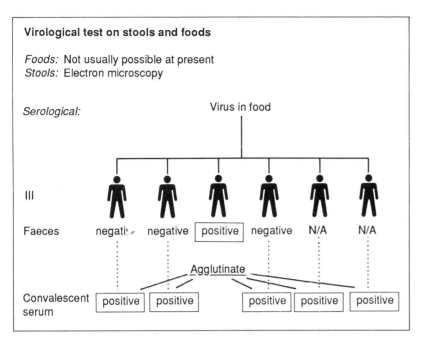

Virological test on stools and foods

Foods: Not usually possible at present
Stools: Electron microscopy

Serological:

Virus in food

III

Faeces   negative   negative   positive   negative   N/A   N/A

Agglutinate

Convalescent   positive   positive   positive   positive   positive
serum

Virological tests on stools and foods—These viruses cannot be grown and are difficult to detect in foods, so laboratories should not be expected to examine foods for them. They can be detected either by electron microscopy in stools while they are being excreted in very large numbers or serologically. Convalescent serum from those affected may agglutinate the virus found in stools.

Clinical features

Salmonellas: Diarrhoea, abdominal pain
Fever, vomiting, septicaemia, localised infections
Staphylococci: **Vomiting,** abdominal pain, diarrhoea, **hypotension**
C perfringens: **Diarrhoea, no fever;** abdominal pain, nausea
V parahaemolyticus: **Profuse diarrhoea,** abdominal pain, vomiting
B cereus – 1: **Vomiting,** nausea, diarrhoea
– 2: **Abdominal pain** and **diarrhoea,** nausea, **no fever**
B licheniformis: **Diarrhoea, vomiting, abdominal pain**
B subtilis: **Vomiting,** diarrhoea, **headache** and **flushing**
E coli: **Cholera like** (ETEC)
Dysentery like (EIEC)
Loose stools/watery diarrhoea (EPEC)
Haemorrhagic colitis, **severe abdominal pain, fever unusual** (EHEC)
Viruses: **Malaise, nausea,** diarrhoea, vomiting, **fever**
Yersinia spp: **Fever, abdominal pain/"appendicitis,"** dysentery like syndrome
Campylobacters: **Bloody diarrhoea** preceded by **fever; abdominal pain,** nausea
C botulinum: Vomiting, **ocular, pharyngeal, respiratory paralysis**
Cryptosporidium: **Prolonged diarrhoea, fever, anorexia, abdominal pain**
L monocytogenes: **septicaemia/meningitis, abortion**
Giardia spp: **Diarrhoea** (acute or chronic), **steatorrhoea,** abdominal pain, **bloating,** weight loss
Scombrotoxin: Diarrhoea, **hot flush, sweating, erythema,** nausea, headache, **palpitations, burning mouth**
Red kidney beans: Nausea, vomiting, diarrhoea
Heavy metals: Nausea, **vomiting,** abdominal pain
Monosodium glutamate: **Burning** and **tightness in chest,** headache, **flushing, thirst,** nausea
Ciguatoxin (dinoflagellates): **Parasthesiae, paresis, respiratory difficulty, dysphagia**
Solanine: **Diarrhoea, vomiting,** headache, **weakness,** abdominal pain, **green stools,** fever, **shock**
Mushrooms: Abdominal pain, vomiting, diarrhoea, **convulsions, coma, hepatorenal failure**

Symptoms and signs in bold are characteristic rather than common.

Although the range of symptoms caused by the common organisms is not great, the type of food poisoning can be suspected from clinical features with fair accuracy. The type of food may also give a clue, although it is wise not to assume too much from this. Food allergy may occasionally cause identical symptoms to those of food poisoning, but skin and respiratory manifestations usually also occur; moreover, food allergy does not occur in outbreaks.

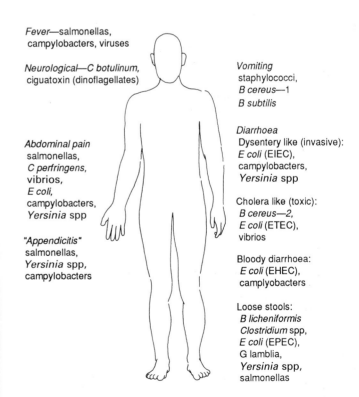

Fever—salmonellas, campylobacters, viruses

Neurological—C botulinum, ciguatoxin (dinoflagellates)

Abdominal pain
salmonellas,
C perfringens,
vibrios,
E coli,
campylobacters,
Yersinia spp

"Appendicitis"
salmonellas,
Yersinia spp,
campylobacters

Vomiting
staphylococci,
B cereus—1
B subtilis

Diarrhoea
Dysentery like (invasive):
E coli (EIEC),
campylobacters,
Yersinia spp

Cholera like (toxic):
B cereus—2,
E coli (ETEC),
vibrios

Bloody diarrhoea:
E coli (EHEC),
camplyobacters

Loose stools:
B licheniformis
Clostridium spp,
E coli (EPEC),
G lamblia,
Yersinia spp,
salmonellas

Food poisoning

Preheated meat (especially casseroles)—*C perfringens, B licheniformis*
Boiled or fried rice, cereals—*B cereus*
Poultry, other meats, eggs—salmonellas
Undercooked poultry—campylobacters
Ham, tongue—staphylococci
Milk and cream—salmonellas, campylobacters, *Yersinia* spp, *Listeria* sp
Cheese—*Listeria* sp, *E coli*, staphylococci

Molluscan shellfish—small round structured viruses
Chocolate—salmonellas
Coconut, dried foods, and spices—salmonellas
Canned food, meat pastes, pies, pasties } staphylococci, *C botulinum, B subtilis, C perfringens*
Seafood—*V parahaemolyticus*

Characteristic type of food—The list here is not comprehensive or mutually exclusive, but may be useful in leading the investigator to suspect certain organisms when the food vehicle is known.

It is not possible to tell from taste or smell or sight that a food is liable to cause food poisoning; the only known exception to this is the uncommon *B subtilis*, when the pie or pasty usually tastes "off."

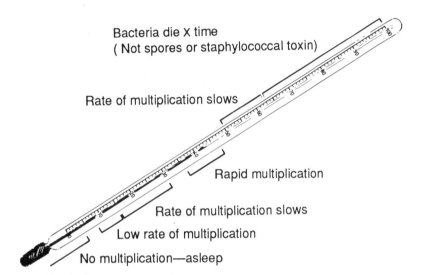

Bacteria die X time
(Not spores or staphylococcal toxin)
Rate of multiplication slows
Rapid multiplication
Rate of multiplication slows
Low rate of multiplication
No multiplication—asleep

Most pathogenic bacteria reproduce fastest (about once every 15–20 minutes) at the body temperatures of humans, 37°C. They do, however, vary slightly in the optimum temperatures. Staphylococci prefer 35–40°C, *B cereus* 28–35°C, and *C perfringens* 43–47°C. Moisture is required for multiplication, but bacteria may survive for long periods in dried foods. Therefore to prevent food poisoning the food should be kept either hot (>63°C), cold (4°C), or dry or otherwise preserved (frozen, pickled, fermented, irradiated, etc). *Listeria* sp and *Yersinia* spp may multiply, albeit slowly, at 4–6°C.

Domestic prevention

Some golden rules
- Defrost thoroughly
- Heat through
- Eat immediately if possible
- Otherwise cool for 1 h
- Refrigerate
- Do not contaminate after cooking

Commonest faults in food preparation
- Cross-contamination—raw to cooked food
- Storage of food at too warm a temperature
- Inadequate cooling
- Storage of food—too long a time
- Reheating—inadequate
- Thawing—inadequate
- Contaminated equipment

More than two faults recorded in more than half of all outbreaks; more than three faults recorded in 17% of all outbreaks.[1]

The following guidelines should be followed:

(1) Heat food thoroughly to kill vegetative cells or pathogenic bacteria. Some organisms, such as *C perfringens* or *B cereus*, will form spores and survive but will remain harmless unless allowed to proliferate by the food being stored in the warmth. It is especially important to heat poultry and boned and rolled meat right through because they are often contaminated (by salmonellas or *C perfringens*) well into the meat. Defrosting such meat and poultry thoroughly is a prerequisite to thorough cooking. If stuffing poultry, weigh it after stuffing to calculate cooking times. Be especially careful with portions of meat over 3 kg (6½ lb).

(2) Eat food within one hour of cooking.

(3) If storage is essential cool as quickly as possible (in less than 1½ hours). A large bulk of food, such as rice, casseroles, discourages rapid cooling, so subdivide it.

(4) Refrigerate at <4°C (check the temperature of the fridge regularly).

(5) For cook-chill, chill to 3°C within 90 minutes of cooking and store at 0–3°C for five days at most, including dates of production and consumption. Detailed Department of Health guidelines are available.

(6) Do not recontaminate food after cooking. Surfaces, utensils, slicers, containers, hands, must be kept entirely separate for raw and cooked foods or washed thoroughly after contact with raw food. Cross contamination may occur in the refrigerator.

(7) When it is being reheated, food must reach boiling temperature throughout. This is obviously easier with small portions of food.

Investigation

Source of infection

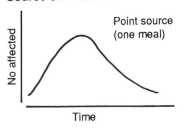

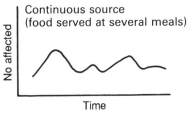

The food handler is rarely the source of infection in outbreaks of food poisoning. Secondary spread occurs only with certain organisms.

Many of the long incubation outbreaks have now been shown to be caused by small round structured viruses. In some outbreaks a cause is still undetectable.

A microbiological diagnosis may be missed because: (*a*) foods are unavailable, or the wrong foods are sent; (*b*) stools are unavailable, the wrong specimens are sent, or the transport conditions are poor; (*c*) the outbreak is notified too late; or (*d*) the laboratory is not given enough detail to look for relevant organisms.

Food contaminated at source

Salmonellas (usually)
C perfringens
V parahaemolyticus } or cross contamination in kitchen
B cereus
Campylobacters

Note:
- Usually waste of time looking for a human carrier source
- Not all salmonella infection is food poisoning

Human carrier

Viruses (faeces)
Staph aureus (skin infections, skin/nasal carriers)
Salmonellas (very rarely) (faeces)

Treatment and prevention

Treatment

(1) No antibiotics if gastrointestinal symptoms only, except metronidazole if symptoms caused by giardia;
(2) Fluids (oral or intravenous) and glucose and salt solutions while diarrhoea is acute;
(3) Antidiarrhoeal agents usually best avoided;
(4) Hygiene must be scrupulous while diarrhoea is acute;
(5) Avoid food handling while diarrhoea is acute.

Prevention

(1) Better food hygiene, both from professional caterers and at home (as above);
(2) Health education for food handlers (red bean poisoning now rare);
(3) Better facilities in kitchens and food storage areas;
(4) Reduce levels of contamination of foods at source—better animal feeding and husbandry, elimination of sources of contamination and opportunities for multiplication of organisms during food manufacturing processes;
(5) Early recognition of outbreaks by appropriate surveillance systems;
(6) Expert investigation of foodborne outbreaks;
(7) Good administration network for withdrawal of contaminated foods (where appropriate) or implementation of other control measures.

Recommendations of the Richmond Committee[2 3]

About 100 recommendations and conclusions are made. They include:

Strengthen surveillance, epidemiological studies, and microbiological studies of components of food chain

Improve coordination between agencies

Create two new committees for:
Microbiolgical safety of food (steering group)
Public health aspects (advisory committee)

Manage outbreaks better (and improve training)

Enforce good manufacturing practice

1 Roberts D. Factors contributing to outbreaks of food poisoning in England and Wales 1970–1979. *J Hyg Camb* 1982;**89**: 491–8.
2 Richmond M. *Microbiological safety of food*. Part 1. Report of the Committee on the Microbiological Safety of Food. London: HMSO, 1990 (Richmond report).
3 Richmond M. *Microbiological safety of food*. Part II. Report of the Committee on the Microbiological Safety of Food. London: HMSO, 1991. (Richmond report).

Norman D Noah is Professor of Public Health and Epidemiology, King's College School of Medicine and Dentistry, London S65 9PJ.
The photomicrograph of small round structured viruses was kindly supplied by Dr E O Caul, Public Health Laboratory, Bristol.
I am grateful to Dr D Roberts for her helpful comments and to John Kramer for information on *Bacillus* spp.

16: FOOD SENSITIVITY

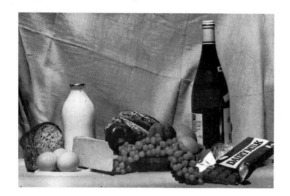

One man's meat is another's poison—LUCRETIUS 96–55 BC

In affluent countries the idea is now widespread that a variety of symptoms (not just those of classical allergy) are caused by individual (hyper)sensitivity to certain foods or substances in them; that such sensitivity has become more common; and that food processing has something to do with it. The media, various unorthodox practitioners, and some groups of lay people have spread the "news". Medical practitioners meanwhile are equipped with little information, most of it confusing, and no reliable diagnostic test to answer their patients' needs.

This is one of the most polarised topics in human nutrition. On one hand many lay people are concerned about sensitivity to food and believe that they suffer from it. On the other hand the medical and food science establishment has been fairly dismissive and declares that most food sensitivity (except adult lactase insufficiency) is rare.

The subject is at the interface between scientific immunology, food technology, and quackery. Good clinical research has been lacking, but recently a few academic departments have started to apply the methods of clinical science to unravel this confusing area. At present it is impossible to give estimates of the objectively confirmed prevalence of most types of sensitivity to food.

Terminology

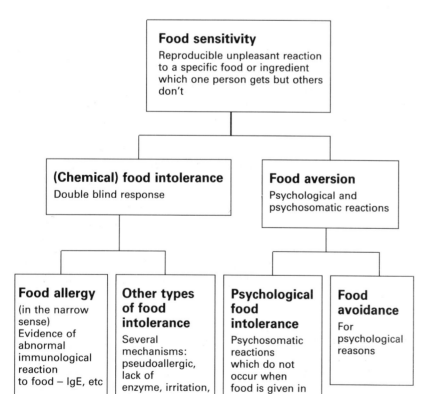

The words describing food sensitivity are imprecise and often used to mean different things.

Food allergy is commonly used by lay people (and by doctors talking to patients) as the broad term, including non-immunological (and sometimes even psychosomatic) reactions. In technical communication the term "allergy" should be confined to immunological reactions.[1-4]

Food sensitivity or *hypersensitivity* is sometimes used in the narrow sense to mean only immunological reactions.

Adverse reaction to food is not used in this chapter because it conveys no meaning of individual susceptibility and includes food poisoning (dealt with in chapter 15).

Pseudoallergic and *anaphylactoid* reactions are used for, for example, asthma or angio-oedema after food with no immunological abnormalities detectable in the patient.

Food idiosyncrasy is used in some classifications for non-allergic food intolerance.

The classification used here is developed from and compatible with the definitions in the report of the Royal College of Physicians.[3]

Diagnosis

Four ways of presentation:
- "Whenever I eat peanuts I get swollen lips, then itchy spots and I sometimes vomit."
- "I can't eat peanuts" (reason why vague or based on a single episode long ago).
- "I wonder if this rash could be caused by something in my diet?"
- "I've given up eating peanuts because the lady in the health food shop (or the lady next door) says I must be allergic to them."

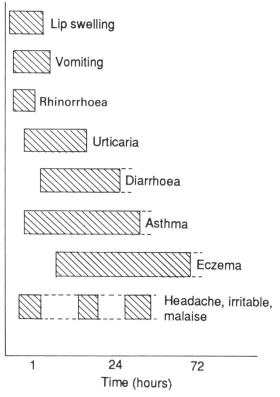

Time course of symptoms of intolerance[1]

Elimination diets

The meat least likely to cause reactions is *lamb*

The least antigenic cereal is *rice*

Vegetables: *peeled potatoes* and *lettuce*

Fruits: *pears* (peeled)

Fat: a refined vegetable *seed oil*, eg (cold pressed) *sunflower* or *safflower*

Drink: *water* and *sugar*

If the diet continues for more than a week an uncoloured multivitamin supplement should be taken.

Other foods are included in some elimination diets, depending on the type of reaction and the suspected ingredients.

Diagnosis of food sensitivity is easy when there is a characteristic early response to a food that is eaten at least occasionally. The patient often notices the association and its reproducibility and tells the doctor the diagnosis.

Diagnosis is more difficult, however, if the clinical reaction is delayed or varies or does not always happen. Such reactions are also made more difficult to judge if someone else has already incriminated a food on circumstantial evidence or because of prejudice.

There are no straightforward diagnostic tests for food sensitivity comparable with the electrocardiogram for coronary disease or the blood urea concentration for renal failure.

Skin tests—Drops of extracts of one or more suspected food antigens are dropped on to the skin and the skin is then pricked or scratched through the drop. A positive response is a wheal and flare within 20 minutes. This indicates the ability of skin mast cells to degranulate in response to the antigen, because they have on their surface IgE specific to the food antigen. Reliability of the test result depends on the quality (specificity) and concentration of the antigen.

The *radioallergosorbent test* (RAST) is a radioimmunoassay performed on serum to show the presence of IgE specific for the food antigen. It is positive in association with IgE mediated food sensitivity.

The skin test and RAST are both sensitive and specific methods for detecting specific IgE, but they do need to be interpreted with care. The *presence* of IgE antibodies to a food does not mean that the patient is *clinically* allergic to it. Many atopic people have IgE antibodies but no symptoms, so positive results must be interpreted in conjunction with a careful history. Foods should not be restricted on the basis of a positive result if no clinical symptoms exist. On the other hand, a negative skin test (or RAST) result is good evidence that a reaction to food is *not* mediated by IgE.

A negative skin test result does not exclude food sensitivity mediated by a mechanism other than the IgE immunological reaction.

Dietary manipulation

The more general diagnostic procedure to indicate food sensitivity is dietary manipulation and recording of symptoms. Such procedures give diagnostic information in food sensitivity of all types. There are several strategies.

Diet diary—The patient or parent keeps a list of all foods eaten and notes any symptoms. This is simple and cheap and can be done at home for several weeks. It is liable to subjective bias, not suitable if the reaction was serious, and difficult to interpret if the responsible agent is present in several foods.

Temporary elimination of one or a few suspected foods—Elimination can be for about a week each time. This is an open trial, liable to subjective bias, but it causes little inconvenience. The method is not suitable if the reaction was serious.

Elimination diet followed by reintroduction of foods one by one—All the foods that commonly provoke sensitivity reactions are eliminated from the diet for two or three weeks. One food is then added back every three to seven days. Elimination diets carry a risk of nutritional deficiency if taken for long or not properly managed.

Patient blind or double blind challenges—After the patient has been stabilised on a standard or elimination diet, foods or ingredients are given in capsules or incorporated into oligoantigenic masking foods. The patient is "blind" to what the foods are. The tests may be carried out in hospital or (more economically but less reliably) at home with the patient recording reactions.

Responses expected with different types of food sensitivity

Type of food sensitivity	Open trial	Blind trial	Immune response
Food allergy	+	+	+
Food intolerance	+	+	−
Psychosomatic	+	−	−
Food aversion	−	−	−

Food sensitivity

Clinical reactions

Food with a high content of natural salicylate include:

dried fruits	many herbs
berry fruits	thyme
oranges	mint
apricots	paprika
pineapples	rosemary
cucumbers	oregano
gherkins	curry
endive	tomato sauce
olives	Worcester sauce
grapes	tea
almonds	wines
liquorice	port
peppermints	liqueurs
honey	

For more details see Swain et al[5]

Foods likely to contain tartrazine (food colour E102) include:

fruit squash	instant puddings
and cordial	coloured sweets
coloured fizzy drinks	filled chocolates
pickles	jelly
bottled sauces	ice cream
salad cream	and lollies
cakes (shop bought)	jam
cake mix	marmalade
soups (packets	curry powder
and tins)	mustard
custard	yoghurt

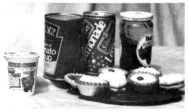

Tartrazine is water soluble and gives a pleasant lemon yellow colour to foods. It is also used in some medicine capsules. Incidence of sensitivity appears to be between 1 in 10 000 and 1 in 1000.

Tartrazine is one of several permitted azo colours. It has been the most tested and incriminated in reactions, but some of the other colours (if eaten in comparable "dosage") might possibly cause reactions in the rare people who are sensitive to tartrazine.

Foods likely to contain sulphur dioxide

Salads in salad bars*
Fresh fruit salad in hotels*
Wines, chilled fruit juices
Pickled onions, dried fruits
Commercial precut chips

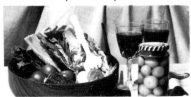

* From "stay fresh" spray

Urticaria and angio-oedema

Urticaria and angio-oedema may be caused by collagen diseases, serum sickness, drug reactions, physical agents, and contact with dusts, among other things. Urticaria may be provoked by foods in four ways.
(1) It may occur as an IgE mediated food allergy, especially to egg (ovalbumin in the white of hen's eggs), peanuts, fish, or cows' milk. These may also cause anaphylaxis.
(2) Large amounts of food which contain histamine releasing agents—for example, strawberries, shellfish, and paw paw—may provoke urticaria.
(3) Foods which contain histamine itself may also provoke urticaria—for example, some wines, fermented cheeses, and sausages. Again, large amounts are needed.
(4) The above foods usually provoke an acute reaction, but chronic urticaria may result from intolerance to salicylates in aspirin and naturally occurring in foods, or to tartrazine, a commonly used yellow food colour, or to benzoates (preservatives in some foods).

Diagnosis of types (1)–(3) is often clear from the history, but in chronic urticaria an elimination diet followed by challenge of aspirin, benzoate, and tartrazine in capsules is necessary to prove the diagnosis. Physical factors—for example, exercise and warmth—tend to cause urticaria on their own and may exacerbate a reaction to food.

Rhinitis and asthma

Foods can precipitate some attacks of asthma in infancy but come well behind infections. The role of foods in asthma diminishes during childhood and they are uncommon precipitants in adults. Inhalants, irritants, infections, pollens and moulds, changes in the weather, and exercise are then all more important. Food sensitivity asthma in adults is largely confined to those exposed to dusty grain, flour, coffee, etc, in their work.

Eggs, seafood, and nuts are among the foods most likely to provoke asthma in children. Skin tests are usually positive, indicating that IgE is implicated, but if the skin test is positive for a food in an asthmatic child, asthma may not follow a double blind challenge. In addition, the response to foods is sometimes psychosomatic.

Patients with aspirin sensitive asthma may benefit from avoiding high salicylate foods. A few cases of asthma induced by monosodium glutamate (E621) have been reported. Whether tartrazine can precipitate asthma now seems doubtful.

The food preservatives sulphur dioxide (SO_2) and sodium metabisulphite can aggravate bronchospasm in established asthmatics. These patients are very sensitive to the irritant effect of SO_2 gas, which is liberated from sodium metabisulphite in acid foods and inhaled in low concentration as the food is swallowed.

Eczema

Infantile eczema and flexural eczema in adults are associated with high serum titres of IgE and often with multipe positive skin tests. In infantile eczema the response to food taking or elimination is slower and less clear cut than in urticaria.

Statistically significant responses to skin tests have been reported in infants apparently sensitive to a food—for example, exacerbation after milk or improvement after withdrawing egg. A controled trial showed improvement in 14 out of 20 children with infantile eczema when egg and milk were removed. Elemental diets (glucose, oil, amino acid mixture, vitamins, and minerals), though expensive, have been helpful in severe infantile eczema. Breast feeding reduces the chance of eczema but only partly in babies with a strong atopic family history. In such cases the mother should avoid eating common allergenic foods.

In adults with eczema a response to elimination diets is less likely. Milk, eggs, and wheat are the most powerful antigens.

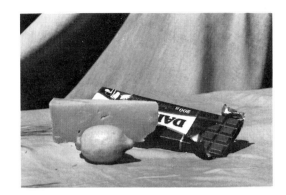

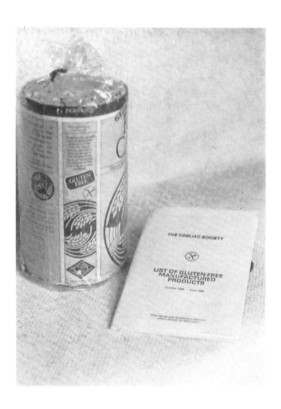

Some less common food sensitivities

Favism—Haemolytic anaemia after eating broad beans. The basic defect is red blood cell glucose-6-phosphate dehydrogenase deficiency.

Bitter lemon purpura—"Bitter lemon" contains quinine, which may rarely precipitate thrombocytopenic purpura.

Chinese restaurant syndrome—As first described, the symptoms were facial pressure, burning sensation in upper trunk and shoulders, and chest pain soon after eating foods rich in monosodium glutamate, particularly Chinese wonton soup. But delayed headache and nausea have subsequently been found to be more common, and asthma has sometimes been precipitated.

Sensitivity to tea or coffee, or both—These common social beverages can cause a variety of pharmacological effects, eg vomiting, headaches, tachycardia, which have sometimes been proved by objective tests.[6]

Migraine

Tension, relaxation, menstruation, bright lights, and hypoglycaemia are among the major precipitants of migraine. Foods can also precipitate attacks. The different factors can be cumulative; several may be needed before an attack occurs. Attacks may come on many hours after a provoking food. Suggestibility and placebo effect have been well established in the responses of migraine sufferers.

Cheese, chocolate, and citrus fruits are often reported to precipitate migraine. They contain pressor amines—tyramine, phenylethylamine, and synephrine, respectively. Alcoholic drinks are another precipitant, notably related to cluster headaches: red wines and some other drinks contain histamine. Other attacks may come about from foods that produce nausea, such as fatty foods. Nitrates, found in some sausages, occasionally cause headaches ("hot dog headache").

True food allergy via IgE is not the usual mechanism in migraine. In a trial in children with severe recurrent migraine at Great Ormond Street most recovered on an exclusion diet. Reintroduction of foods, first "open," later disguised, showed that cows' milk, eggs, chocolate, orange, and wheat were most likely to provoke an attack and tartrazine less commonly.

Gastrointestinal reactions

Many different gastrointestinal sensitivity reactions to food are known and they can act through several different mechanisms. Early symptoms are lip swelling, tingling in the mouth or throat, and vomiting. Later symptoms include diarrhoea, bloating, or even steatorrhoea. Remote symptoms—urticaria, asthma, headache, joint pains—can be associated.

In children immediate intolerance is not uncommon to cows' milk or egg white, nuts, seafood, and some fruits. Tolerance increases with age. Cows' milk allergy can produce a variety of effects, including gastrointestinal bleeding or protein losing enteropathy; eosinophilia may be present.

Coeliac diseae—Sensitivity to wheat gluten is the cause of coeliac disease with jejunal atrophy. It took from 1888, when coeliac disease was classically described, to 1953 before it was found that a fraction of wheat was responsible. A few other foods have been linked with occasional mucosal damage in children, such as cows' milk and soya.

Three month colic occurs at least as often in breast fed as in bottle fed infants. In the former there is no consistent evidence that the colic is related to anything the mother eats.

Irritable bowel syndrome—Evidence for food sensitivity in the irritable bowel syndrome is conflicting. One study, which performed exclusion and double blind challenge, indicated that food sensitivity was common: wheat, dairy foods, maize, some fruits, tea, and coffee were mostly responsible. Another study could not show food sensitivity in most patients.

Intestinal lactase insufficiency is the rule in most adults of Asian and African origin and seen in a minority of white people. There is diarrhoea, abdominal distension, discomfort, and flatus after milk, usually a cupful or more.

Hyperactivity

Feingold in the USA suggested that children (usually boys) with overactivity, short attention span, and impulsive behaviour might improve on a diet which omitted foods containing artificial colours or natural salicylates, or both. Although organisations of parents of difficult children have faith in this hypothesis, objective confirmation is sparse. Most double blind tests with food colours reported significant effects in either none or only one or two of the hyperactive children tested, and some of the information Feingold used on the salicylate content of foods was wrong. Nevertheless, there are some children with a combination of overactivity and physical symptoms (rashes, rhinitis, headaches) suggstive of food sensitivity that have improved on an elimination diet at Great Ormond Street. They appeared on challenge to be sensitive to different foods, but tartrazine and benzoic acid were top of the list.

Food sensitivity

1 Lessof MH, ed. *Clinical reactions to food.* Chichester: John Wiley, 1983.
2 Marabou Symposium. Food sensitivity. *Nutrition Reviews* 1984;**42**:65–139.
3 Royal College of Physicians and the British Nutrition Foundation. Food intolerance and food aversion. *J R Coll Physicians London* 1984;**18**:2.
4 American Academy of Allergy and Immunology Committee on Adverse Reactions to Foods. National Institute of Allergy and Infectious Diseases. *Adverse reactions to food.* Bethesda, Md: National Institutes of Health, 1984. (NIH Publication No 84-2442.)
5 Swain AR, Dutton SP, Truswell AS. Salicylates in foods. *J Am Diet Assoc* 1985;**85**:950–60.
6 Finn R, Cohen HN. "Food allergy": fact or fiction? *Lancet* 1978;i:426–8.
7 Panush RS. Nutritional therapy for rheumatic diseases. *Ann Intern Med* 1987;**106**:619–21.
8 Pearson DJ. Pseudo food allergy. *BMJ* 1986;**292**:221–2.

Further reading

Lessof MH. Adverse reactions to food additives. *J R Coll Physicians London* 1987;**21**:237–40.
Young E, Patel S, Stoneham M, *et al.* The prevalence of reaction to food additives in a survey population. *J R Coll Physicians London* 1987;**21**:1–7.
Kjeldsen-Kragh J, Haugen M, Borchgrevink CF, Laerum E, Eck M, *et al.* Controlled trial of fasting and one-year vegetarian diet in rheumatoid arthritis. *Lancet* 1991;**338**:899–902.

Arthritis

Gouty arthritis is aggravated by alcohol and by high purine and high protein diets. Although most patients with rheumatoid arthritis do not respond to food exclusions or challenges, a patient whose arthritis was clearly shown to be aggravated by milk and cheese was reported from the Hammersmith Hospital. A small minority of similarly reacting rheumatoid patients was found in a subsequent study in Florida.[7]

Pseudo food allergy[8]

Apparent reactions to food are quite often psychological rather than organic in origin. Patients may be convinced, but on circumstantial or no real evidence, that they are sensitive to certain foods. These beliefs are encouraged by some popular books and unorthodox practitioners, and are not easy for the busy general practitioner to change. Avoiding a broad range of foods carries a risk of malnutrition. Parents have also been reported as having inflicted supposed allergies on their children—a variant of Meadow's syndrome.

Specialist food "allergy" (sensitivity) clinics are available at some of the teaching hospitals, such as Addenbrooks, Cambridge; Great Ormond Street, London; Guy's, London; etc.

17: PROCESSING FOOD

STEWART TRUSWELL AND JANETTE BRAND MILLER

In the guessing game, "Animal, vegetable, or mineral?" nearly all foods are animal or vegetable or the two combined. What we eat is other organisms, some of them—fruits and cereals—still viable. The basic material of our foods has an anatomy and a histology. It is made of cells which contain numerous enzymes and biochemical compounds that are the same as or similar to those in the human body. Foods are also inhabited by micro-organisms. These multiply after slaughter or harvesting and nearly all our basic foodstuffs deteriorate rapidly because of autolytic decay and microbial activity. Foods can become dangerous because of these unless we treat them in some way. Cereal grains are the major exception. They have a low water content and normally keep for years when dry at ambient temperatures. The major early civilisations were built on this property, and even today the only staple foods that are kept in savings banks are the cereals.

Insect activity also leads to appreciable losses of food.

> • "Doctors need to know as much about foods as they do about drugs."
>
> • "Each medical school should have an expert on the biochemistry of foods among their preclinical lecturers."
>
> *Two recommendations from the Interntional Union of Nutritional Sciences Workshop on Nutrition Education for Medical Practitioners,* held at the Royal College of Physicians, London, *March 1984.*[1]

Why foods have to be processed or prepared

> ### Food technology
>
> *Handling after harvest*—Foods must be kept at the best temperature, atmosphere, etc, between the farm and market or factory.
>
> *Food processing* is treatment of food in a plant or factory before it is sold in the shop.
>
> *Food preparation* is treatment of food in the kitchen, at home, in a catering establishment or take away shop. It is a wider term than "cooking", which implies the use of heat.
>
> Between each treatment stage food has to be *stored*; the conditions affect how long it keeps and its quality.

(1) Foods are preserved so that they can be kept for longer. Preservation reduces wastage and hence cost. It enables people in affluent communities to eat their favourite foods all the year round and also enables us to benefit from economies of scale by growing large quantities of a food on large areas of suitable land. Preservation also helps to feed the growing world population.

(2) Processing or preparation makes foods safe to eat by destroying or retarding the growth of pathogenic micro-organisms (such as salmonella, clostridia, or fungi) or inactivating natural toxins (such as trypsin inhibitors and goitrogens).

(3) Processing or preparation improves the attractiveness of food, its flavour, and its appearance. This is not a frivolous function. Poorly prepared food is often the chief complaint of patients in hospitals and nursing homes.

(4) Processing also provides convenience. In Mrs Beaton's time most women spent their lives working for hours each day in the kitchen. Modern convenience foods have liberated women in countries like Britain. Much of the work that used to be done by hand in the Victorian kitchen is now done by machines, some controlled by computer, in the food processing plant or factory.

Methods of food preservation and processing

> Some of the most important processes used for our foods go back to the stone age.
>
> • The Sumerians had a simple dairy industry. Butter is mentioned several times in the Bible (eg *Isaiah* vii, 15).
>
> • The ancient Egyptians brewed beer and discovered how to make raised bread. Beer has been called "liquid bread."

Drying—Traditionally this was sun drying or smoking, but nowadays tunnel drying, spray drying, and freeze drying produce concentrated forms of the foods—for example, milk powder or coffee powder. Bacteria, which require water, cannot grow and autolytic enzymes are inhibited.

Freezing prevents bacterial growth because bacterial enzyme activity slows then stops as temperature is lowered. In addition, water in the food is not in an available form.

Addition of salt or sugar is a third way of lowering the "water activity" and preventing bacterial growth, just as sugar has been shown to reduce infection in wounds.

Heat is used in several ways. Blanching (1–8 min at 100°C depending on the food) before freezing and canning inactivates enzymes that would otherwise continue autolysis of the food. Pasteurisation of milk (72°C for 15 seconds) destroys pathogenic organisms but not others. Cooking destroys all or nearly all organisms (except spore formers depending on conditions). Sterilisation of canned and other sealed foods is performed by subjecting the food to a high temperature with or without pressure.

Processing food

Nutrients per 100 g in wholemeal (100%) and white [breadmaking] (72%) wheat flour

Nutrients	Wholemeal	White
Energy kJ (kcal)	1318 (314)	1451 (346)
Protein (g)	12·7	11·5
Fat (g)	2·2	1·4
Starch (g)	62	74
Sugars (g)	2·1	1·4
Dietary fibre (g)	8·6	3·7
Thiamin (mg)	0·47	0·32*
Riboflavin (mg)	0·09	0·03
Niacin (mg)	5·7	2·0*
Vitamin B-6 (mg)	0·5	0·15
Total folate (μg)	57	31
Vitamin E (mg)	1·4	0·3
Iron (mg)	3·9	2·1*
Zinc (mg)	2·9	0·9
Calcium (mg)	38	140*
Total phosphorus (mg)	320	120
Phytate phosphorus (mg)	240	30

* As fortified in the United Kingdom.

Food irradiation is a new technique useful for replacing ethylene oxide in sterilising spices (whose flavour would change on heating). It can also extend the shelf life of strawberries and mushrooms, inhibit sprouting of potatoes, and destroy pathogens on poultry.[2]

Refrigeration does not destroy micro-organisms but those present cannot multiply or do so only slowly; it also slows autolysis by enzymes in the food.

Fermentation produces acid or ethanol, or both, which inhibit pathogenic and spoilage organisms.

Chemical preservatives—Benzoic acid, propionic acid, and sorbic acid, naturally present in cranberries, Gruyère cheese, and rowanberries, respectively, are added to certain specified foods in controlled amounts to prevent bacterial growth. Sodium metabisulphite, which liberates sulphur dioxide in the food, is used for the same purpose.

Packaging—Once a food has been heat sterilised reinfection is prevented by sealing it in a can or airtight plastic bag or multilayer paper or plastic carton. Packaging of unsterilised food, though not preventing bacterial growth, reduces contamination and prevents loss of water through evaporation, etc.

Separation methods—Unlike the methods above these are not used to preserve foods. Milling produces different fractions of cereal flours. Pressing produces oils from oil seeds and juice from fruit.

Fresh or processed?

Most "fresh" fruit in the greengrocers comes from overseas or has been stored for weeks or months. "Fresh" vegetables too, though mostly home grown, are often stored. Bananas are picked in the tropics before they are ripe, shipped and stored at a controlled even temperature ($>13°C$), and ripened by exposure to ethylene gas (which is given off naturally by ripening fruit). Oranges are picked ripe, shipped, and stored at a lower temperature ($3°C$) in dry air with a raised carbon dioxide level. The skins have to be protected from mould infection, for example, by wrapping with chemically impregnated paper. Although these fruits have been in artificial environments, they are intact and alive and their cells are absorbing oxygen and producing carbon dioxide.

Likewise, it is worth money to understand what factors determine tenderness and flavour in meat. There is a speciality of meat science, which shares some of the histological and biochemical knowledge used by clinicians who specialise in muscular diseases.[4] Before slaughter animals should have adequate muscle glycogen. This is converted to lactic acid, which acts as a weak preservative. Fresh meat is tough because of rigor mortis. This disperses during hanging in a controlled temperature of $-1·4°C$—that is, chilled not frozen.

Food additives

Salt, vinegar, nitrates, and sugar have been used for centuries and are still among the most used food preservatives today. Hops are a traditional preservative for beer. Many of history's great voyages of exploration were made in search of food additives. Marco Polo journeyed to the East to obtain exotic spices. Cortez brought back vanilla from the Aztecs.

Preservatives are permitted in specified foods at concentrations up to a maximum—for example, nitrates in bacon and ham, sulphur dioxide in dried fruit, propionic acid in bread.

Antioxidants are used to prevent the slow oxidation of oils and fats by atmospheric oxygen and development of rancidity. Concentrations and types in different foods are regulated.

Emulsifiers keep oil and aqueous phase together in sauces. Lecithin is an example.

Humectants prevent foods from drying out. Glycerol is an example.

Foods acids are acids that occur naturally. They are used for flavour or for technical reasons—for example, to adjust the pH in certain jams so that the pectin sets—and can also act as preservatives.

Anti-caking agents stop lumps forming in powdery foods.

Thickeners may be vegetable gums, cellulose derivatives, or starch derivatives.

Humectants	
Glycerol	E422
Sorbitol	E420
Food acids	
Acetic acid	E260
Citric acid	E330
Malic acid	E296
Anti-caking agents	
Calcium hydroxy phosphate	E341
Magnesium carbonate	E504
Thickeners	
Guar gum	E412
Locust bean gum	E410
Pectin	E440
Carboxymethyl-cellulose	E466
Colours–natural	
Beetroot red	E162
Carbon black	E153
Chlorophyll	E140
β carotene	E160(a)
Colours—synthetic	
Tartrazine	E102
Brown FK	154
Erythrosine	E127
Flavour enhancers	
Monosodium glutamate	E621
Sodium inosinate	E631

Additives with code numbers that do not have the E prefix are controlled by the UK but not yet by the European Commission (EC).

Nutritional supplements are now given by name on the label. A number of foods are fortified or enriched with nutrients—for example, margarine includes vitamins A and D, flour and bread and some breakfast cereals contain some B vitamins, and textured vegetable proteins contain vitamin B-12.

Colours—Only a few colours are permitted in the European Community. Half of them are natural—for example, beetroot red, carbon black, chlorophyll, and various carotenoids. Synthetic colours are a short list mostly of azo dyes, but erythrosine is an iodine compound.

Miscellaneous—Other additives include enzymes like rennin, bleaching agents, firming agents, antifoaming agents, phosphates, surfactants, propellants for aerosol food containers, and air excluders.

Flavours—The Council of Europe has listed over 2000 flavouring substances which may be added to foods, normally in minute quantities and without hazard to public health. The names of individual flavours are not declared on labels and they are not included in the E code, but use of flavourings is included among the ingredients. Flavour recipes in foods are trade secrets. Most flavours are naturally derived by distilling or extracting the essential oils. Others are synthetic but chemically identical with one of the characteristic flavour compounds that have been identified in foods—for example, citral, the chief flavour ingredient of lemon oil. A small but growing group of artificial (non-caloric) sweeteners is permitted in foods in Britain: these include saccharin, aspartame, and acesulfame K.

Contaminants

Unintentional additives can get into foods somewhere along the chain from farm to plate. Examples are pesticides, other farm chemicals, drugs, heavy metals (lead, cadmium, mercury, and arsenic), industrial chemicals—for example, polycyclic aromatic hydrocarbons and polychlorinated biphenyls, atmospheric and water pollutants, radioisotopes, and phthalate plasticisers. Foods are monitored for most of these by government agencies, such as the Ministry of Agriculture, Fisheries, and Food as part of a continuing surveillance programme.[5]

Are our foods safe?

Potentially toxic substances in foods

Natural

Inherent, naturally occurring	Usually present in the food and affect everyone if they eat enough, eg solanine in potatoes.
Toxin resulting from abnormal conditions of animal or plant used food	Eg neurotoxic mussel poisoning; honey from bees feeding on rhododendron nectar.
Consumer abnormally sensitive	Eg coeliac disease from wheat gluten; allergy to particular food; or drug induced, eg cheese reaction.
Contamination by pathogenic bacteria	Acute illness, usually gatrointestinal eg infection with *Salmonella* spp or campylobacters or toxins produced by *Staphylococcus aureus* or *Clostridium botulinum* (food may not appear spoiled).
Mycotoxins	Food mouldy or spoiled, eg aflatoxin B_1 from *Aspergillus flavus* is a liver carcinogen.

Manmade

Unintentional additives—manmade chemicals used in agriculture and animal husbandry	Eg, fungicides on grain, insecticides on fruit, antibiotics or hormones given to animals.
Environmental pollution	Eg, organic mercury, cadmium, polychlorinated biphenyls, and radioactive fallout can affect any stage of food chain.
Intentional food additives: preservatives, emulsifiers, flavours, colours, etc	The most thoroughly tested and monitored of all chemicals in food.

Britain had the first food safety legislation in the world, the Sale of Food and Drugs Act 1875; this and subsequent acts have been replaced by the Food Act 1984. An expert committee, the Food Advisory Committee, advises the Minister of Agriculture, Fisheries, and Food and the Department of Health. Its reports are distributed for comments by industry, consumers, and scientists and then may be developed into regulations under the Act. A new committee, the Advisory Committee on Novel Foods and Processes, advises on new foods and processes (eg food irradiation) and the impact of biotechnology.

These expert committees are in regular informal communication with the EC Scientific Committee for Food, the Joint FAO/WHO Expert Committee on Food Additives, and food toxicologists round the world.

Deliberate food additives are not intrinsically toxic substances. They have been tested in several animal species and are kept under review continuously by food toxicologists.

Processing food

Amounts permitted in foods are such that the maximum intake does not exceed the acceptable daily intake (usually 1/100 the highest level that has no effect in animal tests). Toxicological tests have not so far systematically examined the chances of hypersensitivity reactions in man, and such occasional reactions to tartrazine, sulphur dioxide, and monosodium glutamate are described in chapter 16.

Sir Richard Doll estimates that whereas various components in the diet account for around 35% of deaths from cancer, food additives account for only 1% and some may even be protective. There is a greater potential risk to health from other substances in foods.

Losses of nutrients

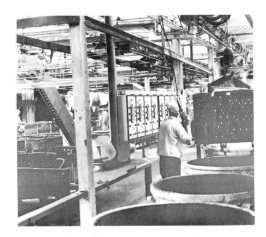

Some losses of nutrients occur during food processing but they are qualitatively and quantitatively similar to the losses that happen in domestic cooking. Most processes in the food factory are scaled up versions of one or other home recipe. Factory processes are standardised and controlled but home cooking varies from excellent to bad. Nutrient losses are roughly predictable and can easily be measured by analysis at different stages.

Two vitamins are more unstable than the others when heated, vitamin C and folate, but whereas vitamin C lasts better in acid medium, folate does not. Thiamin (vitamin B_1) is moderately unstable when heated. Riboflavin decomposes in ultraviolet light. Water soluble vitamins dissolve into the cooking water and the more water used the more vitamins are likely to be wasted. Mineral nutrients are stable but can also be washed out if large amounts of cooking water are used. Lysine, the limiting amino acid in cereals, is the most unstable of the essential amino acids. The golden crust of bread is coloured by a complex of sugars and lysine which becomes biologically unavailable. There is some loss of linoleic acid in oils when they are reused for frying, especially at high temperatures.

Losses of vitamin C are worth considering in detail. The factors that cause the oxidative breakdown of vitamin C are tissue damage (which liberates ascorbic acid oxidase) by bruising or freezing of leafy vegetables, heating in alkaline water—for example, with sodium bicarbonate added—contact with copper, and leaching into the processing or cooking water. Moderate losses occur between harvesting and

Percentage retention of vitamin C in peas after different stages of preparation (after Mapson[6])

Fresh	Frozen	Canned	Air dried
—	Blanching 75	Blanching 70	Blanching 75
—	Freezing 75	Canning 63	Drying 45
—	Thawing 71	Diffusion 40	—
Cooking 44	Cooking 39	Heating 36	Cooking 25

Effect of different conditions on stability of nutrients in foods (based on Harris and Karmas[7])

Nutrients	Effect of solutions			Effect of exposure to			Cooking losses (% range)
	Acid	Neutral	Alkaline	Oxygen	Light	Heat	
Vitamins							
Vitamin A	U	S	S	U	U	U	0– 40
Vitamin D		S	U	U	U	U	0– 40
Vitamin E	S	S	S	U	U	U	0– 55
Thiamin	S	U	U	U	S	U	0– 80
Riboflavin	S	S	U	S	U	U	0– 60
Niacin	S	S	S	S	S	S	0– 50
Folate	U	U	S	U	U	U	0– 80
Vitamin C	S	U	U	U	U	U	0–100
Amino acids							
Leucine, isoleucine, methionine, valine, and phenylalanine	S	S	S	S	S	S	0– 10
Lysine	S	S	S	S	S	U	0– 40
Tryptophan	U	S	S	S	U	S	0– 15
Threonine	U	S	U	S	S	U	0– 20
Mineral salts	S	S	S	S	S	S	0– 3

U = Unstable, S = Stable.

	Vitamin C (mg/100 g)
729 **Peas**, raw	24
730 **Peas**, boiled	16
731 **Peas**, frozen, boiled	12
733 **Peas**, canned, reheated	1
725 **Mange-tout** peas, boiled	28
726 **Mange-tout** peas, stir-fried in oil	51

From *McCance and Widdowson's The Composition of Foods*, 5th ed[8]

cooking fresh vegetables and when a bottle of fruit juice is opened and kept at room temperature. There is little difference in losses of vitamin C between three methods of cooking: boiling, microwave, and pressure cooking, but the less water used the less vitamin is thrown away in the water. There are substantial losses of vitamin C when cooked vegetables are kept warm before they are served or refrigerated until the next day.

On average losses of vitamin C in cooking may be taken as 70%—that is, 30% retention—in leafy vegetables and 40% in root vegetables. Food tables usually give values for cooked vegetables which allow for this as well as for the raw food.

Perspective

Last century cows were kept in towns because there was no way of preventing milk from souring. To provide the milk, cheese, yoghurt, and cream for the people of London about 0·5 million cows are needed. They in turn each need about 7 acres of farm land to feed them through the year. From these 3·5 million acres scattered across the south of England fresh milk is pooled, transported, pasteurised, bottled, and distributed or processed in other ways. Other foods—fruits, meat, fish in Britain—may come from half way around the world. This complex movement and distribution of foods would be impossible without food processing.

(1) Some loss of nutrients is inevitable in food processing, but for most nutrients losses are small.

(2) Manufacturing losses, when they occur, are often in place of similar losses through cooking at home.

(3) The importance of the losses in a particular food has to be considered in relation to the whole diet. If a food makes only a small contribution to the intake of nutrients processing losses are not of practical importance. On the other hand, changes in any food that makes a major contribution to nutrient supply—for example, milk for babies and cereals in some adults—need continued vigilance.

(4) There are some beneficial effects: destruction of trypsin inhibitor in legumes and liberation of bound niacin in cereals. Nutrient enrichment is possible.

(5) Other advantages of food processing are protection from pathogenic organisms, better flavour, and cheaper price. Often the ultimate choice is between dried, canned, or frozen peas (say) in late winter or no peas at all.

1 Truswell AS, (rapporteur). Nutrition education for medical students and practitioners: report of a workshop. *UN University Food and Nutrition Bulletin* 1984;**6**:75–81.

2 Truswell AS. Food irradiation. (Editorial) *BMJ* 1987;**294**:1437–8.

3 Holland B, Unwin ID, Buss DH. *Cereals and cereal products*. Third supplement to *McCance and Widdowson's the composition of foods*. (4th ed.) Cambridge: Royal Society of Chemistry, 1988.

4 Lawrie RA. *Meat science*. 4th ed. Oxford: Pergamon, 1985.

5 *Food surveillance: a description of the Government's extensive surveillance and reporting of nutrients and chemicals in our food*. London: Ministry of Agriculture, Fisheries, and Food, 1989;1–28. (PB0025.)

6 Mapson LW. Effect of processing on the vitamin content of foods. *Br Med Bull* 1956;**12**:73–7.

7 Harris RS, Karmas E. *Nutritional evaluation of food processing*. 2nd ed. Westport, Connecticut: Avi, 1975.

8 Holland B, Welch AA, Unwin ID, Buss DA, Paul AA, Southgate DAT. *McCance and Widdowson's the composition of foods*. 5th ed. Cambridge: Royal Society of Chemistry, 1991.

Further reading

Food additives: the balanced approach. London: Ministry of Agriculture, Fisheries, and Food, 1987:1–28. (PB0037.)
(Booklet explaining how to read ingredient lists in food labels, giving code numbers and uses of additives.)

Look at the label. London: Ministry of Agriculture, Fisheries, and Food, 1988: 1–29. (PB0038.)

Pesticides and food: a balanced view. London: Ministry of Agriculture, Fisheries, and Food, 1989:1–13. (UB63.)
(All three booklets available from Food Sense, London SE99 7TT or HMSO bookshops.)

We thank K J Dale of the Ministry of Agriculture, Fisheries, and Food for his helpful comments.

18: SOME PRINCIPLES

There are two questions affecting health about any food.
(1) Is it safe, or will it harm me (*a*) immediately or (*b*) later if I eat it repeatedly?
(2) Is it good for me?

Is it "food"?

For a food one has not eaten before question 1*a* predominates. If it has not been contaminated or infected the answer depends ultimately on folklore. In every culture there are parts of plants and animals that the group recognises as food which other cultures do not. Only a minority of plants can be expected to be freely edible. For most plants it would be an evolutionary advantage to possess a toxin that discourages animals from eating it. Our folklore about which plants are edible comes down from unknown ancestors who took the risk of eating an unfamiliar plant, sometimes with unfortunate results.

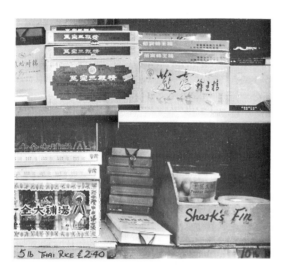

Is this food good for me?

Simple trial and error by people with primitive technology cannot answer questions 1*b* or 2. One of the difficulties for professionals who give advice about healthy diets is that there is no immediate symptom of well being corresponding to the surge of amino acids or vitamins that blood samples can show. The feelings of satiety and of inner warmth after a meal are much the same after a good nutritious one as after a meal that contains only "empty calories". One rare exception is the gratifying faecal result that occurs within hours of eating wheat bran in people inclined to constipation. This is probably why the fibre hypothesis was accepted by lay people years before it was well supported by human experiments. The only reliable way to answer questions 1*b* and 2 is by the methods of nutritional science.

Origins of our scientific knowledge about human nutrition

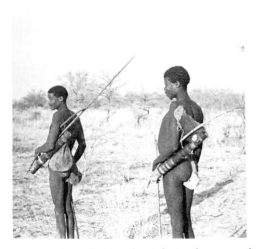

Hunter-gatherers in general were lean and ate more plant than animal foods, though they did eat meat or seafoods. They ate a variety of foods, had a high fibre intake, but took no salt or alcohol and concentrated sugar only rarely (as wild honey). The photograph shows contemporary hunters, two !Kung bushmen in the northern Kalahari, Botswana (taken by the author in 1968).

- *Comparative and evolutionary*—Homo sapiens and his predecessors have been on the earth one million years or more. Ninety nine per cent of this time our ancestors lived as hunter-gatherers. Agriculture started only 10 000 years ago. There has not been enough time for our species to evolve any new mechanisms required by the recent food supply. Natural selection, which must work chiefly via reproductive success, has been distorted by inequality of wealth and lately by technology. It is difficult to see how it could modify diseases that start in middle age. But presumably our bodies have evolved well adapted for doing what hunter-gatherers did and eating what they ate. We have information from archaeological records and from studies of the few fast disappearing groups of contemporary hunter-gatherers.[1 2]

- *Experiments of nature and travellers' tales*—From people who eat different foods from us, under stable conditions or during a disaster, we can form hypotheses about the physiological effects of different food patterns that we could not easily persuade our fellow countrymen to adopt. We have, for example, learnt about the physiological role of very long chain polyunsaturated fatty acids from the Eskimos,[3] and about deficiency diseases from nutritional experiences of prisoners of war.[4]

- *Epidemiological studies* range in the power of their design. Associations and correlations of disease characteristics and dietary variables do not prove cause and effect, but prospective studies, especially if repeated in different groups, give valuable information on the relation between usual diets and chronic diseases.[5]

Some principles

Some examples of human experiments and trials

• Intervention trial of low saturated fat diet in half of 850 middle aged male veterans in Los Angeles over five years

• Trials of vitamin C against placebo for preventing colds during winter

• Experimental depletion of a single nutrient in human volunteers

• Long term testing of the value of novel protein foods

• Experiments measuring energy expenditure

• Metabolic balance studies—for example, to assess the effect of diet on plasma cholesterol

• Absorption and uptake studies—for example, glycaemic index after different foods containing carbohydrates

• *Animal experiments* were the principal technique for working out the vitamins.[6] The right animal model has to be used. Understanding of scurvy was static and controversial until Norwegian workers found (in 1910) that guinea pigs are susceptible like man because, unlike most animals, they cannot synthesise ascorbic acid from glucose.

• *Clinical records* have been informative about the role of diet in disease, including inborn errors of metabolism. Information about requirements for trace elements has come recently from experiences with total parenteral nutrition.[7]

• *Food analysis*—The independent variables in nutritional epidemiology and in dietetic treatment of disease are food constituents. Food analysis is work that is never finished; foods keep changing and demand develops for constituents not measured before, such as different types of dietary fibre and fatty acids C20:5 and C22:6. To facilitate international sharing of what food composition data there is INFOODS (the International Network of Food Data Systems) was set up in 1983.

• *Human experiments and trials* last from hours to years and many different variables can be measured (see box).

The three groups of substances in foods

(1) *Energy and nutrients*

Man needs oxygen, water and enough food energy (calories), 10 or more indispensable amino acids in proteins, essential fatty acids—for example, linoleic acid—a small amount of carbohydrate, 13 vitamins, and 18 elements scattered across the upper half of the periodic table (in addition to hydrogen, carbon, nitrogen, and oxygen).

Together they add up to over 40 nutrients, many of which are normally taken for granted: the minor nutrients are present in sufficient amounts in a mixed diet of foods. But for long term total parenteral nutrition all the minor vitamins and trace elements must be included in the required postabsorptive amounts.

For some of the nutrients *you can have too much of a good thing.* Generous intakes of saturated fat raise the plasma cholesterol concentration and contribute to coronary heart disease. People with high salt intakes have more hypertension. Too much food energy leads to obesity.

The three groups of substances in the edible portion of foods

Energy and nutrients
Water and packing
Other substances
Colour, flavouring, etc.
Natural non-nutritive substances, "xenobiotics", some of which are potential (or even established) toxins.

(2) *Water and packing*

All foods contain water. In many it is more than half the weight. The percentage of water is higher in some fruits and vegetables than in milk. The more water a food contains, the fewer calories. But this water has to be counted in the diet of patients with anuria. The "packing" of plant foods—that is, dietary fibre—is not all inert. Some fractions have physiological effects: arabinoxylans (hemicelluloses) of wheat increase faecal bulk and speed colonic transit; pectins slow absorption of lipids and glucose.

(3) *All the rest and toxins*

All the many other substances in foods are non-nutritive. They produce most of the flavour, colour, and other sensory qualities. In most natural foods there are inherent

Size of adult requirements for different nutrients

Adult daily requirement in foods	Essential nutrients for man
2–10 µg	Vitamin D, Vitamin B-12, Cr
c 50 µg	Vitamin K, Se
c 100 µg	Biotin, I
200 µg	Folate, Mo
1–2 mg	Vitamin A, thiamin, riboflavin, vitamin B-6, F, Cu
c 5 mg	Mn, pantothenate
c 15 mg	Niacin, vitamin E, Zn, Fe
c 50 mg	Vitamin C
300 mg	Mg
c 1 g	Ca, P
1–5 g	Na, Cl, K, essential fatty acids
c 50 g	Protein (10 or more essential amino acids)
50–100 g	Available carbohydrate
1 kg (l)	Water

Figures are approximate and in places rounded. The range of requirements for different nutrients is about 1000 million.

Some principles

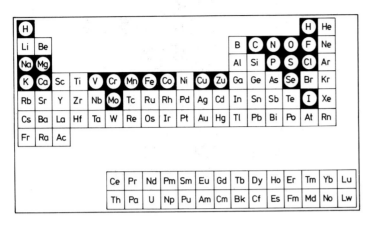

Periodic table of the elements. Those essential for man are blocked in. Vanadium is provisional. In addition, Ni, Si, and traces of As have been shown to be essential in some animals. Boron has been reported to reduce urinary calcium loss in women.[8]

substances that are potentially toxic but usually present in small amounts—for example, solanine in potatoes, nitrates and oxalates in spinach, thyroid antagonists in brassica vegetables, cyanogenetic glycosides in cassava and apricot stones, etc. Then there are substances that only some people are sensitive to—for example, in some people wheat causes gluten enteropathy, broad beans favism, and cheese a tyramine effect in patients taking monoamine oxidase inhibitors.

Other toxins get into foods when their environment is unusual—for example, toxic shellfish after a "red tide"—or if polluted with industrial contaminants, such as methyl mercury, polychlorinated biphenyls, etc. Microbiological infection can produce very potent toxins, such as botulism and aflatoxin. Deliberate food additives are not known to be toxic—if they were they would not be permitted by international or national food administrations. A few can cause sensitivity reactions in a minority of people (see chapter 16 on food sensitivity).

Patterns of nutrients in different foods

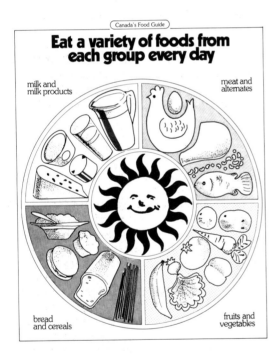

If animals are fed only one food sooner or later they will become ill and die. No single food contains all the essential nutrients. Wheat (wholemeal flour) lacks vitamins A, B-12, C, and D and is very low in iron and calcium (if unfortified); beef contains little or no calcium, vitamins A, C, or D, or dietary fibre. On the other hand, wheat is a good source of dietary fibre and beef of iron and vitamin B-12. The two together provide more nutrients than either alone but between them have no vitamin C or D and hardly any calcium. Addition of citrus fruit or salad brings vitamin C into the mixture, and milk or cheese adds the missing calcium and a little vitamin D.

This is the theory behind the "basic four" food groups for educating the public about nutrition. Each group has some deficiencies which the other three make up between them. You should aim to eat more than one serving each day from each of: the bread and and cereals group; the meat, poultry, and fish group; the vegetable and fruit group; and the milk group.

Variety

It is not enough to have daily servings of the same food from each group. One should choose a variety within food groups for two reasons. Firstly, the characteristic nutrients in each group vary greatly for individual foods. Among fruits the vitamin C ranges from negligible (for dried fruits, raw pears, and figs) up to 140 to 150 mg/100 g for stewed blackcurrants and canned guavas (this is in the British food tables; the international range goes up to about 3000 mg/100 g).[9]

Secondly, natural toxins do not follow any of our arbitrary groupings of foods. The wider the variety of individual foods that people eat, the less their chance of acquiring harmful amounts of the toxins that are inevitable in foods but usually in small and subclinical amounts.

Blending dietary guidelines with food groups

The four groups are intended to minimise deficiency of traditional nutrients—protein, calcium, vitamin C, etc. In affluent countries, however, more disease is probably caused by too much fat, salt, and alcohol and not enough carbohydrate or fibre. So we have to modify the older message. In Holland each of their four food groups is now subdivided into first preference and second preference subgroups, based on the amounts of fat, sugar, and fibre in individual foods.

Possible modifications of four food groups to incorporate dietary guidelines

- *Bread*—Yes but wholegrain and with lower salt. Prefer lower fat, low salt *cakes* and *biscuits*.
- *Meat*—Lean cuts with the fat removed and not fried. Alternate with *fish* (grilled) and *legumes*.
- *Vegetables* slightly cooked, not with salt.
- *Fruit* fresh, not canned in syrup or dried.
- *Milk* with half or all the cream removed.

Average nutrient density of milk and milk products

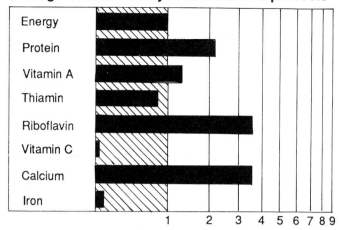

Average nutirent density of meat group

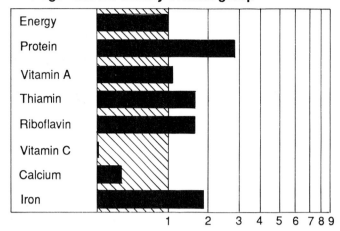

Average nutrient density of fruit and vegetables

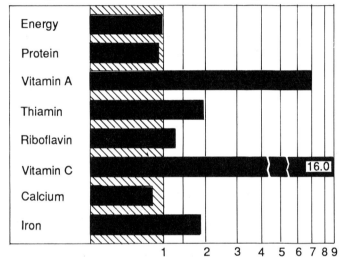

Nutrient density is the ratio of a nutrient (expressed as % of recommended daily intake) to energy (expressed as % of a standard energy intake). In the total diet of mixed foods the density for each nutrient should exceed 1·0. (From Hansen RG.[10])

Junk foods and nutritious foods

Whether a food is nutritionally bad or good depends on the rest of the diet. As Hippocrates taught, "All things in nutriment are good or bad relatively." An extra portion of saturated fat is bad in Britain but would be good for starving children in north east Africa. An orange does nothing for someone who takes vitamin C tablets but is important for an elderly person who eats no vegetables. Value judgments about foods are being made all the time; they are nearly always subjective and usually wrong.

A good objective method is to work out for a typical serving of the food its provision of important nutrients as a percentage of their recommended dietary intakes compared with its content of energy (calories), also as a percentage of a standard daily intake. For each nutrient

$$\text{the index of nutritional quality} = \frac{\text{nutrient as \% standard}}{\text{energy as \% standard}}$$

The profile of indices for major nutrients can be put in an array. Other components in the food, like cholesterol, saturated fatty acids, and dietary fibre can be treated in a similar way by using a dietary goal as the standard.

The example, modified from an American book,[11] shows that egg contains a smaller proportion of fat per enegy (calories) than butter; the fat is less saturated and egg is also a good source of protein and some other nutrients. Egg and butter both contain some vitamin A but this is the only essential nutrient (other than a tiny amount of linoleic acid) in butter. However, an egg contains much more cholesterol than $\frac{1}{2}$ oz butter.

Calculations of this type should be made before authorities advise whole communities to eat more or less of a food. Applying them to the 1984 DHSS recommendations[12] about diet to prevent cardiovascular disease means that the amount of butter eaten should be reduced more than the amount of egg, because reduced saturated fat is recommended but current cholesterol intake is not considered excessive. In the United States, however, a dietary guideline advises against high levels of dietary cholesterol (see p 29) and so recommends the general public to moderate its consumption of egg yolks.

Indices of nutritional quality (INQ) for butter and egg

	Butter ($\frac{1}{2}$ oz; 14 g)			Egg (50 g), hard boiled		
	Amount	% Of standard	INQ	Amount	% Of standard	INQ
Energy (kcal)	100	5	1·0	80	4	1·0
Vitamin A (mg)	0·129	11	2·2	0·078	7	1·6
Thiamin (mg)	0	0	0	0·04	4	1·0
Riboflavin (mg)	0	0	0	0·14	12	2·9
Niacin (mg)	0	0	0	0·03	0	0
Vitamin C (mg)	0	0	0	0	0	0
Iron (mg)	0	0	0	1·0	6	1·5
Calcium (mg)	3	0	0·07	28·0	3	0·8
Potassium (mg)	4	0	0·02	65	1	0·3
Protein (g)	0	0	0	6	12	3·0
Carbohydrate (g)	0	0	0	1	0	0·1
Fat (g)	12	15	3·1	6	8	1·9
Oleic acid (g)*	2·9	12	2·4	2	8	2·0
Linoleic acid (g)	0·3	2	0·3	0·6	3	0·8
Saturated fatty acids (g)*	7·2	25	5·1	1·7	6	1·5
Cholesterol (mg)*	32	11	2·2	225	75	19

Based on Hansen RG *et al*.[11] [The standards they used are energy 2000 kcal (8·4 MJ), vitamin A 1·2 mg, thiamin 1 mg, vitamin C 60 mg, riboflavin 1·2 mg, niacin 14 mg, iron 16 mg, calcium 900 mg, potassium 5000 mg, protein 50 g, carbohydrate 275 g, fat 78 g, oleic acid 24·5 g, linoleic acid 20 g, saturated fatty acids 28·5 g.] I have taken 300 mg as standard for cholesterol.
*Not essential nutrients.

Some principles

Energy values as metabolised in the body of the main energy-yielding groups of food components (Atwater factors)

	kcal/g	kJ/g
Fat	9	37
Alcohol	7	29
Protein	4	17
Carbohydrate*	3·75	16

*This is for available carbohydrate. The energy provided by dietary fibre from its fermentation to volatile fatty acids in the large intestine is less than half this amount.

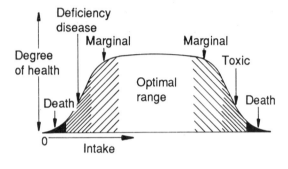

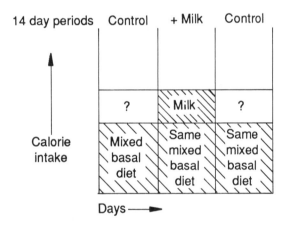

Calories do count

The law of conservation of energy applies to human nutrition as in the rest of nature. Atwater established this around 1900. A little more heat may be produced after some foods or in some people but the more calories (or kilojoules) you eat the more you can expect to store as adipose tissue.

Foods differ in their calorie content from 29 kJ/100 g (7 kcal/100 g) for boiled French beans, cabbage, celery, and vegetable marrow up to 3·8 MJ/100 g (899 kcal/100 g) for vegetable oils—a 128-fold range. This great range depends on the different energy values of fat, alcohol, protein, and carbohydrate and how much these are diluted by water. It is useful for doctors to know the energy values of average servings of common foods (there is a short list in chapter 11 on obesity).

No perfect diet

There are several diets that appear (in our present state of knowledge) to be good. We can advise on a better diet for Mr Smith or, as in a US report, make recommendations "Towards healthful diets," but there is no best diet. The reason is that man is an omnivore with enzyme systems that can adapt to ranges of intakes of many food components. There is, for example, an inducible enzyme sucrase in the small intestinal epithelium; if people eat sucrose this enzyme appears and digests it. There are several enzymes in the liver which oxidise proteins; their activity increases when protein intake is high and falls in people on low protein diets.

When the intake of one nutrient is varied and the rest of the diet is held constant there is a middle range, over which health does not improve or deteriorate as the intake is changed. For most nutrients this is quite a long range. There is therefore no single optimal intake figure. The recommended dietary intake or reference nutrient intake is intended to be at the top of the left hand slope in the diagram.

Replacement

For every food you remove from the diet another has to take its place. This principle is prominent in the design and interpretation of nutritional experiments. Does consumption of milk raise or lower the plasma cholesterol concentration? To test this an adequate but physiological amount of milk is to be given in a middle two or three week period and the plasma cholesterol value measured at the end of this period and at the end of equal length control periods before and after. But what should be given to replace the calories of the milk in the control periods? If nothing is given the periods will not be isocaloric.

To some extent the effect of milk on plasma cholesterol could be manipulated by the choice of the control food. We do not want to influence the experiment so might ask, "If people here stop drinking milk what would they drink (or eat) in its place: beer, water, fruit juice, fizzy drink, etc?" A similar situation applies in outpatients when the doctor or dietitian instructs a patient to cut out one food from his diet. Unless he is to lose weight he will sooner or later choose other food(s) as replacement, which may affect the outcome.

Some concluding proverbs

People have been thinking about the safety and goodness of food as well as its social roles and tastiness ever since the Garden of Eden or its evolutionary counterpart. So it is perhaps not surprising that a number of proverbs about food and eating are being confirmed by nutritional science.

Moderation in all things—The recommendation of many expert committees on nutrition. Don't eat too much or too little of anything and don't follow one of the extreme unorthodox regimens.

Variety is the spice of life—You should eat a mixed and varied choice of foods.

Enough is as good as a feast—More leads to obesity. People's energy requirements differ. "Enough" is an individual amount.

You can have too much of a good thing—For example, saturated fat, salt, dietary cholesterol, vitamins A, D, and B-6 and alcohol.

One man's meat is another man's poison—The subject of chapter 16 on food sensitivity. For each of us there are foods we dislike and may well be foods that can make us ill.

There's no accounting for taste—Taste has to be considered in planning therapeutic diets.

A little of what you fancy does you good—Dietary prescriptions are sometimes more rigid than they need be. This proverb also speaks of the placebo effect: if someone believes a food is doing him good he may feel better for a time after eating it.

Old habits die hard—Food habits must be respected.

Prescribed dietary changes are likely to be followed better if they are fitted into the least strongly held of an individual's food habits.

There's many a slip twixt cup and lip—People don't necessarily eat what they intend or say they eat. That patient you just put on a diabetic diet may not have understood you.

1 Truswell AS, Hansen JDL. Medical research among the !Kung. In: Lee RB, DeVore I, eds. *Kalahari hunter-gatherers*. Cambridge, Massachusetts: Harvard University Press, 1976.

2 Eaton SB, Konner M. Paleolithic nutrition. A consideration of its nature and current implications. *N Engl J Med* 1985;**312**:283–9.

3 Leaf A, Weber PC. Cardiovascular effects of n-3 fatty acids. *N Engl J Med* 1988;**318**:549–57.

4 de Wardener HE, Lennox B. Cerebral beriberi (Wernicke's encephalopathy). *Lancet* 1947;i:11–7.

5 Shekelle RB, Shyrock AM, Paul O, *et al*. Diet, serum cholesterol and death from coronary heat disease. The western electric study. *N Engl J Med* 1981;**304**:65–70.

6 Widdowson EM. Animals in the service of human nutrition. In: Taylor TG, Jenkins NG, eds. *Proceedings of the XIII International Congress of Nutrition* (Brighton, 1985). London: John Libby, 1986: 52–7.

7 Freund H, Atamian S, Fischer JE. Chromium deficiency during total parenteral nutrition. *JAMA* 1979;**241**:496–8.

8 Nielsen FH, Hunt CD, Mullen LM, *et al*. Effect of dietary boron on mineral, estrogen and testosterone metabolism in postmenopausal women. *FASEB J* 1987;**1**:394–7.

9 Brand JC, Cherikoff V, Lee A, Truswell AS. An outstanding food source of vitamin C. *Lancet* 1982;ii:873.

10 Hansen RG. An index of food quality. *Nutr Rev* 1973;**31**:1–7.

11 Hansen RG, Wyse BW, Sorenson AW. *Nutritional quality index of foods*. Westport, Connecticut: Avi Press, 1979.

12 Department of Health and Social Security. *Diet and cardiovascular disease*. (Report of the panel on diet in relation to cardiovascular disease, Committee on Medical Aspects of Food Policy). London: HMSO, 1984.